FITNESS FOR LIFE

Middle School

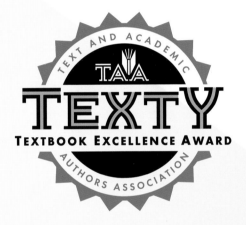

Charles B. Corbin

Guy C. Le Masurier

Dolly D. Lambdin

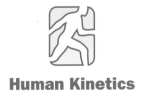

Human Kinetics

Library of Congress Cataloging-in-Publication Data

Corbin, Charles B.
  Fitness for life : middle school / Charles B. Corbin, Guy C. Le Masurier, Dolly D.
Lambdin.
      p. cm.
  Includes bibliographical references and index.
  ISBN-13: 978-0-7360-6511-5 (hard cover)
  ISBN-10: 0-7360-6511-3 (hard cover)
  1. Exercise--Physiological aspects. 2. Physical fitness for youth. 3. Exercise for youth.
I. Le Masurier, Guy C. II. Lambdin, Dolly, 1951- III. Title.
  RJ133.C665 2007
  613.7'10835--dc22
                                  2007000958

ISBN-10: 0-7360-6511-3
ISBN-13: 978-0-7360-6511-5

The Web addresses cited in this text were current as of December 2006, unless otherwise noted.

The illustration on the back cover is adapted, by permission, from C. Corbin and R. Lindsey, 2005, *Fitness for life*, 5th ed. (Champaign, IL: Human Kinetics), 64.

Acquisitions Editor: Scott Wikgren; **Developmental Editor:** Ray Vallese; **Assistant Editor:** Derek Campbell; **Copyeditor:** Patsy Fortney; **Proofreader:** Joanna Hatzopoulos Portman; **Indexer:** Ann Truesdale; **Permission Manager:** Dalene Reeder; **Graphic Designer:** Robert Reuther; **Graphic Artist:** Angela K. Snyder; **Photo Manager:** Laura Fitch; **Art/Photo Office Assistant:** Jason Allen ; **Cover Designer:** Robert Reuther; **Photographers (cover):** Kelly Huff, Tom Roberts, © Image 100 LDT; **Photographers (interior):** © Human Kinetics, unless otherwise noted; © Getty Images (pp. 7, 42 [top right and bottom left], 56 [second and third photos]); © Photodisc (pp. 18, 42 [top left], 56 [far right], 68 [top left and bottom right], 83 [left], 97 [top], and 108); courtesy of Charmain Sutherland (p. 29); © Image Source (pp. 30 and 104); courtesy of Chuck Corbin (p. 34); © Brand X Pictures (p. 52); courtesy of Scott Wikgren (pp. 57 [top] and 59 [top left]); © Stockdisc (p. 92); **Art Manager:** Kelly Hendren; **Illustrators:** Argosy, unless otherwise noted; art on pp. 4, 28, 40, 53, 66, 80, 96, 99 and the back cover by Mic Greenberg and Al Wilborn; **Printer:** Custom Color Graphics

Printed in the United States of America   10 9 8 7 6 5 4

Human Kinetics
Web site: www.HumanKinetics.com

United States: Human Kinetics
P.O. Box 5076
Champaign, IL 61825-5076
800-747-4457
e-mail: humank@hkusa.com

Canada: Human Kinetics
475 Devonshire Road, Unit 100
Windsor, ON N8Y 2L5
800-465-7301 (in Canada only)
e-mail: info@hkcanada.com

Europe: Human Kinetics
107 Bradford Road
Stanningley
Leeds LS28 6AT, United Kingdom
+44 (0)113 255 5665
e-mail: hk@hkeurope.com

Australia: Human Kinetics
57A Price Avenue
Lower Mitcham, South Australia 5062
08 8372 0999
e-mail: info@hkaustralia.com

New Zealand: Human Kinetics
Division of Sports Distributors NZ Ltd.
P.O. Box 300 226 Albany
North Shore City, Auckland
0064 9 448 1207
e-mail: info@humankinetics.co.nz

contents

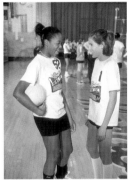
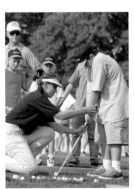
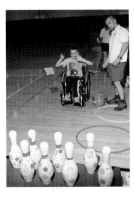

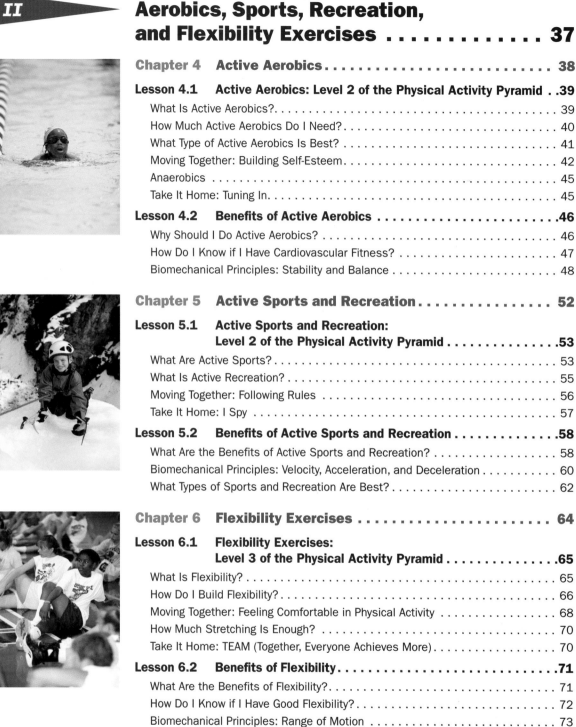

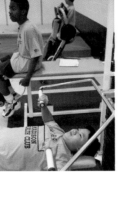
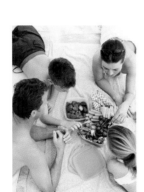
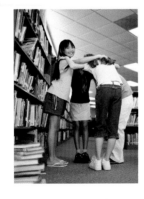

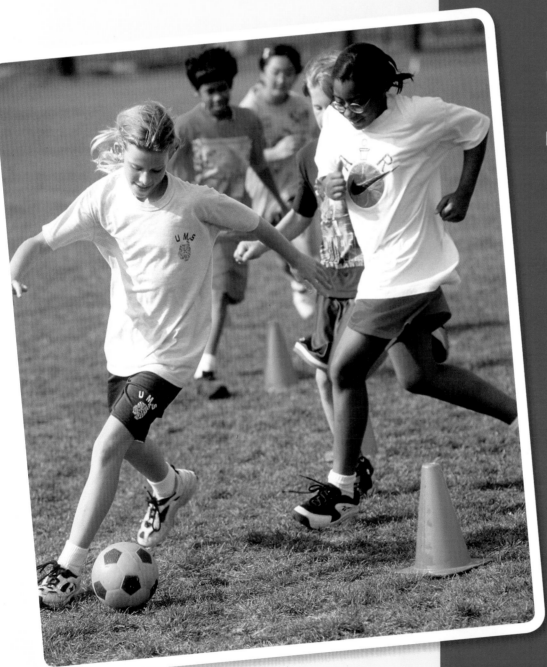

Touring *Fitness for Life: Middle School*

Do you want to be healthy and fit? Do you want to look your best and feel good? *Fitness for Life: Middle School* will help you meet your fitness and physical activity goals. Take this guided tour to learn about all of the features of this textbook.

The *Fitness for Life: Middle School* program includes several other components:

▶ **Teacher's Guide.** Your teacher has a special *Teacher's Guide* with lessons and activities that you can do to better learn and understand the information in this textbook.

▶ **Worksheets and Resources.** Special worksheets guide you in putting the information to use in assignments and projects.

▶ **Web Site.** The *Fitness for Life: Middle School* Web site (www.fitnessforlife.org/middleschool) offers further information on topics involving fitness and physical activity.

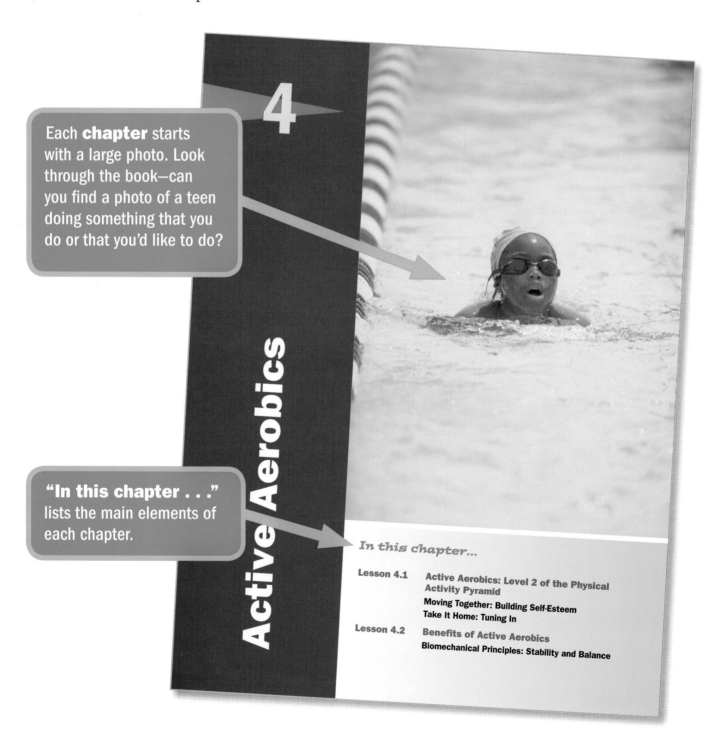

Each **chapter** starts with a large photo. Look through the book—can you find a photo of a teen doing something that you do or that you'd like to do?

"**In this chapter . . .**" lists the main elements of each chapter.

4

Active Aerobics

In this chapter...

Lesson 4.1   Active Aerobics: Level 2 of the Physical Activity Pyramid

Moving Together: Building Self-Esteem
Take It Home: Tuning In

Lesson 4.2   Benefits of Active Aerobics
Biomechanical Principles: Stability and Balance

Lesson vocabulary lists the key terms in each lesson. These terms appear in bold type the first time they're used in the lesson. They're also defined in the book's glossary and on the *Fitness for Life: Middle School* Web site.

Fit Facts offer interesting facts about health and fitness.

Opening questions describe the **objectives** of each lesson to show you what you'll learn.

Visit the *Fitness for Life: Middle School* **Web site** for extra information about topics. Go to www. fitnessforlife.org/ middleschool, click on "Student Information," and click on the topic number.

Lesson **5.2**

Benefits of Active Sports and Recreation

Lesson Vocabulary
acceleration, deceleration, velocity

Click Student Info ▸ Topic 5.6

When you participate in active sports and recreation, you get health, wellness, and fitness benefits. Can you describe some of the most beneficial active sport and recreation activities? What are some of the best types of sports and recreation for you? When you finish this lesson, you'll know the answers to these questions. You'll also understand the importance of acceleration and velocity to your performance in physical activity.

What Are the Benefits of Active Sports and Recreation?

Sports have many benefits. Perhaps the best benefit is that they're fun. Even if you don't enjoy all sports, you probably have found several that you do enjoy. Even the least active sports and recreation activities provide health benefits similar to those provided by lifestyle physical activities. Active sports and active recreation have the added advantage of building cardiovascular fitness. This is one reason why active sports and recreation are included along with active aerobics in level 2 of the Physical Activity Pyramid. To gain cardiovascular fitness, you must follow the FIT formula that you learned in chapter 3. You must perform active sports and recreation for at least 20 minutes at least three days a week, and your heart rate must be elevated into the target heart rate zone.

Sports and recreational activities can help you in many other ways as well. They can help you to relax and reduce the stresses in your life. They cause your body to expend calories that can help you maintain a desirable weight and feel and look your best. They provide a great way to meet friends and enjoy social interactions. They can help you learn to work as part of a team, which can benefit you in your adult career. Finally, participation in active sports and recreation can help you build parts of fitness other than cardiovascular fitness, including flexibility and muscle fitness. You'll learn more about these in later chapters.

Use the worksheet supplied by your teacher to interview other students about their favorite active sports and recreation activity. Ask them about the fitness benefits they gain, why they enjoy the activity, and what advice they can give to others who want to try the activity.

Click Student Info ▸ Topic 5.7

FIT FACT

Sports and recreation activities can be adapted for people with disabilities. In "beep-beep softball," the ball makes a beeping noise so that people who are visually impaired can participate. In wheelchair tennis, a person in a wheelchair is allowed two bounces to get to the ball.

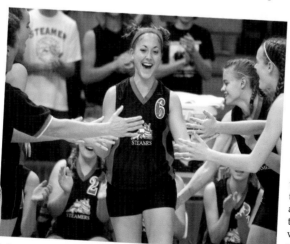
Active sports provide a way to meet friends and enjoy social interactions.

Fitness for Life: Middle School

Each chapter has a **Moving Together** feature that helps you learn how to have fun with others in many different kinds of activities.

Each Moving Together presents a **situation** in which teens have to deal with a certain problem.

Questions let you come up with ways for the teens to solve the problem.

Guidelines for problem solving offer suggestions for helping teens.

Moving Together: Full Participation

Can you remember a time when you were the leader of a group in a physical activity setting? How did you perform as a leader? Were you successful at getting all members of your group to participate? What strategies did you use to promote participation? How do you feel when people don't pay attention to you? How do you feel when some members of a group do less work than others?

Jimmy and Molly were in physical education class. The class was doing an exercise routine that required them to try several different skills and then do them to music. They were assigned to a group to read about a skill and then show the class how to do it properly. Molly was the group leader. She read the directions for the skill, showed the group a picture of it, and asked all group members to try it.

When it was her group's turn, Molly was going to read the class a description of the skill and have all group members demonstrate at the same time. But some group members didn't pay attention. Two group members were talking about other things. Jimmy just quietly stood to the side.

Discussion Questions

1. What could Molly do to get all group members to participate in the activity?
2. How could Jimmy help Molly to keep the group working together?
3. What other suggestions do you have to help the group complete its assignment?
4. Are there any other questions we should ask?

Guidelines for Full Participation

Everybody learns faster and better when all members of a group are actively involved in the group activity. Two kinds of guidelines can help the group to have full participation: group leader guidelines and group member guidelines.

Click Student Info ▶ Topic 2.4

If you're the leader of a group, follow these guidelines.

▶ *Use basic leadership skills.* These include things such as speaking with a strong voice, maintaining eye contact when you talk to other group members, and showing enthusiasm for what you're doing.

▶ *Ask questions of the group members.* By asking questions of others in the group, you increase the participation by all group members.

▶ *Ask group members to help demonstrate skills.* You can show your enthusiasm by demonstrating some of the skills yourself, but you can also involve others in the group by asking them to demonstrate skills.

▶ *Have all group members practice the skill together.* If group members practice the skill with you, they may feel more involved in the group's activity.

▶ *Give positive feedback to those who try.* Thank them for their effort.

▶ *Tell group members that it is OK to make a mistake.* We all make mistakes at first. Practice will help everyone improve.

If you're asked to participate as a member of a group, follow these guidelines.

▶ *Help the leader by participating.* In this class all students will get a chance to be a group leader. When you're the leader, you'll want the help of other students, so giving your help when you're a group member will help get the cooperation of others when you're the leader.

▶ *Avoid talking when the leader is talking.* This is one of the best ways to help the leader. Also, paying close attention to the leader will help you learn the skill the leader is teaching.

▶ *Give your best effort in all activities.* Effort is one of the most important factors in learning. Most people don't succeed the first time. If you get in the habit of working you can do all skills hard at first.

"Bio" comes from "biology," and "mechanical" is a word that describes machines. So the **Biomechanical Principles** feature in each chapter helps you learn to use your body—the human machine—in physical activity.

The bold sentence summarizes the **key point** of the principle.

Study and **apply the principle** described in the feature.

Follow these suggestions to put the **principle in practice** and see how it works for you.

Biomechanical Principles: Energy, Force, and Movement

Energy and force are necessary for producing human movement.

Energy means "available power." We use electric power to provide energy to light our houses and to power appliances such as television sets and washing machines. Electric companies provide the energy using coal, gas, oil, wind, or nuclear sources. The food you eat provides the energy that allows your muscles to contract. When your muscles contract, they produce **force** that causes the bones to move, creating movement of body parts and total body movement. For example, when the muscles of your legs contract, your legs move. Leg movement allows you to move the whole body, such as when you walk.

You move most efficiently when the force produced by the muscles is applied in the direction in which you want to move. For example, when you throw a ball, it's best to apply force to the ball by moving your arm in the direction you want the ball to go. The more force the muscles apply, the farther the ball will travel. Also, the longer the force is applied, the more force you can apply. If you reach back a long way before throwing the ball, you can apply force forward for a longer time, and you can throw the ball farther. When you walk or run and do other movements, the same rules apply.

Sir Isaac Newton is credited with developing three laws of motion. These laws are related to force and how it's used to create and regulate motion. Much of the information provided here is based on Newton's laws. For more information about force and Newton's laws relating to force, visit the *Fitness for Life: Mi[...] School* Web site.

Click Student Info ▶ Topic 1.8

Applying the Principle

To move well, you need to know how to use force efficiently and effectively. In walking and running, f[...] example, it's best to appl[...] [...]e force in line with the d[...]tion of movement. Ex[...]s have discovered sev[...] rules that will help yo[...]e the force that your [...] produce when pushin[...] the ground.

▶ Point your feet and toes straight ahead (see photo below left), not to the side (see photo below right). This allows the force from your legs and feet to keep you moving forward and doesn't waste force to one side or the other.

▶ Swing your arms in line with the direction of the intended movement to avoid wasting force. Swinging your arms to the side reduces the forward force that you can produce with your legs.

▶ Avoid twisting your body. Keep your trunk (hips, belly, and chest) facing the direction you are walking or running.

▶ Apply force for the full time that your foot is on the ground. When you are in the air (such as in running) no force can be applied and so you can't increase your speed.

▶ To move faster, apply more force. Fast walking and running will require you to apply more force than slow walking.

Principle in Practice

Correct application of force is important for efficient and effective movement in normal daily activities and in physical activities of all kinds. Work with a partner to see if you're applying force properly when walking and running. Have your partner watch your arms and legs to see whether your movements are straight ahead or to the sides. If your movements include motion to the sides, try to change the way you walk or run to be more efficient.

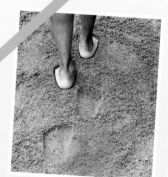

Good force application.

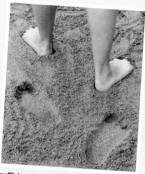

Inefficient force application.

Do I Need Supplements?

Teens who want to build muscle fitness sometimes want fast results. They may think that the answer is to take **supplements** with long names that promise to build fitness and increase performance. The Food and Drug Administration (FDA), a government agency that regulates foods and drugs, defines a supplement as "a product taken by mouth that contains a 'dietary ingredient' intended to supplement the diet." Supplements are different from medicines. Medicines must be approved by the FDA before they can be sold, but the FDA doesn't have to test and approve supplements. Supplements include vitamins, minerals, herbs, proteins, and many other substances. They're found in many forms such as tablets, capsules, gelcaps, liquids, or powders and bars that look similar to candy bars.

Eating good food and performing regular muscle fitness exercise is the best way to build muscle fitness. Supplements are costly and unnecessary, and they might contain substances other than what are listed on the package. Because supplements aren't regulated by the government, there's no guarantee that you're getting what you think you're getting when you buy a supplement. You should also know that supplements can cause side effects or unwanted negative problems including headaches, dehydration, changes in heartbeat, and allergies. The people who advertise supplements rarely warn you of the side effects. You should consider supplements only when your doctor has recommended them and your parent or guardian approves.

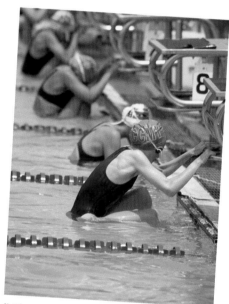

Holding the body still before the start of a race requires isometric strength.

Take It Home

Building Muscle and Character

Strength can be displayed in many ways. Physical strength is needed for rock climbing and cheerleading. In this chapter you learned how to build muscles to improve physical strength. Mental strength is tested during a chess match. You learn how to improve mental strength in many of the classes you take in school.

Strength of character is another kind of strength. It's tested daily, and it defines you as a person. Are you honest? Do you play fair? Do you take responsibility for your own actions? Do you stand up for others even when it's the unpopular thing to do? Do you respect others regardless of their age, gender, and ethnic background? Are you a caring person? Are you a good citizen in your class, neighborhood, community, and country? Your answers to these and other questions indicate your strength of character.

Use the worksheet supplied by your teacher to show how you can demonstrate strength of character in physical education.

Lesson Review

▸ What is muscle fitness?

▸ Describe the overload principle and the principle of progression, and explain how they're important to muscle fitness development.

▸ Define the terms isotonic exercise and isometric exercise, and give examples of each type of exercise.

▸ Describe the FIT formulas for building strength and muscular endurance.

▸ Describe several guidelines for performing muscle fitness exercises safely.

▸ Do you need supplements to build muscle fitness?

▸ Describe some guidelines for preventing bullying in physical activity settings.

> The **Chapter Review** section at the end of each chapter helps you reinforce what you've learned.

6

Chapter Review

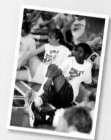

Number your paper from 1 to 5. Read each question. After the number for the question, write a word or a phrase that best answers the question. The page number where you can find the answer is listed after the question.

1. What term describes the amount of movement in a joint? (page 65)
2. What word describes tissue that connects bone to bone? (page 66)
3. What is another word used in this chapter to describe static or nonmoving? (page 66)
4. How many seconds should you hold each static stretch of a muscle to get the best benefits? (page 70)
5. What health problem associated with poor flexibility adults at some time in their lives? (page 71)

Number your paper from 6 to 10. Next to each number, best answer.

6. gravity
7. tendon
8. back-saver sit-and-reach
9. strain
10. hypermobility

a. one aid in producing a
b. an injury to a muscle
c. tissue that connects n
d. a test of flexibility
e. too much range of mot

> If you have questions about what you've learned in each chapter, you can **Ask the Authors** at the *Fitness for Life: Middle School* Web site.

> A **Unit Review** is provided at the end of each group of three chapters. After you complete each unit, visit the Web site to review what you've learned and try to solve a puzzle of fitness terms.

Number your paper from 11 to 15. Follow the direct question or statement.

11. Explain the difference between a static stretch and PNI
12. Give three or more examples of static stretching exercises
13. Give three or more examples of guidelines for feeling more comfortable in physical activity.
14. Give three or more examples of the health benefits of good flexibility.
15. Give examples of the normal range of motion for two different joints.

Ask the Authors

When is the best time to do stretching exercises to improve flexibility?

Get the answer and ask your own questions at the *Fitness for Life: Middle School* Web site.

Click Student Info ▶ Topic 6.10

Unit Review on the Web

You can find unit II review materials on the *Fitness for Life: Middle School* Web site.

Click Student Info ▶ Topic 6.11

editorial board

Unit I

Fitness and Activity for All

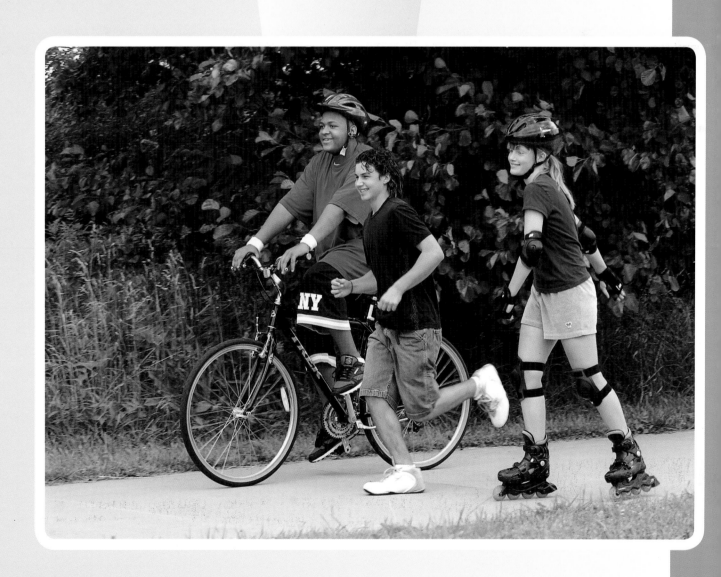

Introduction to Physical Activity and Fitness

1

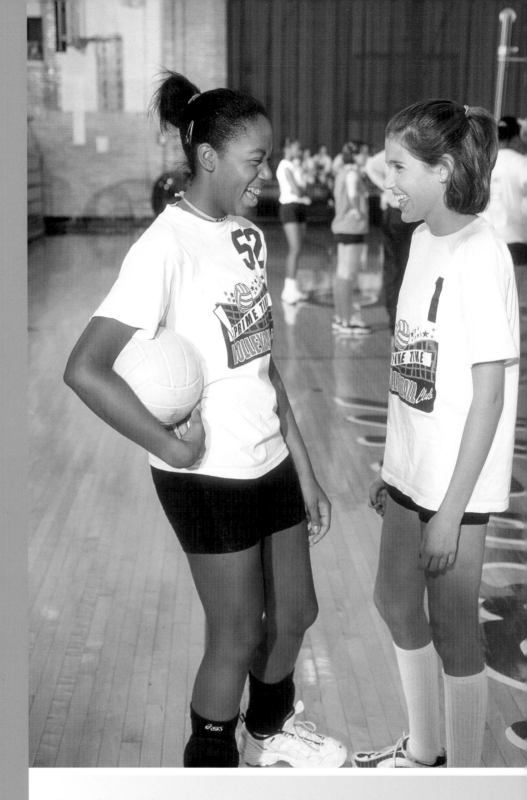

In this chapter...

Introduction to Physical Activity

Lesson Vocabulary

active aerobics, active recreation, active sports, aerobic, cool-down, exercise, flexibility exercises, lifestyle physical activities, lifetime activities, moderate activities, muscle, muscle fitness exercises, physical activity, vigorous activities, warm-up

▶ **www.fitnessforlife.org/middleschool/**

Click Student Info ▶ Topic 1.1

Like most teens, you probably know that you need to be physically active. But do you know why? Do you know what types of activities are best for you? When you finish this lesson, you'll know the answers to these questions. You'll also know more about good communication so that you understand what other people are saying and so that they understand what you mean.

What Is Physical Activity?

Physical activity occurs when your muscles contract to make your body move. Experts recommend that teens spend at least 60 minutes and up to several hours performing physical activity each day. The Physical Activity Pyramid for teens (see page 4) shows many types of physical activity from which you can choose. Ideally you would choose activities from each of the first three levels of the pyramid. You can combine activities from all three levels to meet the daily activity recommendation.

The activities at the bottom (first level) of the pyramid are called **lifestyle physical activities** because you do them as part of your daily life. Examples include walking to school, working around the house, and working in the yard. These physically beneficial lifestyle activities are called **moderate activities** because the intensity is not too easy and not too hard. Experts recommend that adults do moderate

physical activity for 30 minutes or more each day. This is because activities from level 1 of the Physical Activity Pyramid help people reduce their risk of disease and help them maintain a healthy body weight. As you'll learn later in this book, it's recommended that teens do regular moderate activity to get the same benefits as adults and to develop activity habits that can last a lifetime.

Lifestyle and other moderate activities are sometimes called **lifetime activities** because you can do them when you're young as well as when you grow older. Some activities from other levels of the pyramid are also considered to be lifestyle or lifetime activities. For example, certain sports such as bowling and golf and certain recreational activities such as fishing can be included in level 1 of the pyramid because they're moderate in intensity. They can be considered lifetime activities because they can be done by people of all ages.

Activities at the second level of the teen pyramid include active aerobics and active sports and recreation. These activities are good for building physical fitness, especially cardiovascular fitness. They also provide health benefits similar to those of moderate lifestyle activities. The activities at the second level of the pyramid are considered **vigorous activities** because you use more energy doing these activities than you use when doing moderate lifestyle activities. Experts recommend that teenagers do these vigorous activities at least three days a week for 20 minutes. These activities make your heart beat faster and make you breathe faster than normal. Active sports and recreation activities, such as tennis and dancing, and active aerobics, such as aerobic dance, are considered to be lifetime activities because many people of all ages perform them.

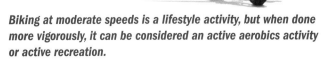

Biking at moderate speeds is a lifestyle activity, but when done more vigorously, it can be considered an active aerobics activity or active recreation.

Active aerobics is a type of vigorous physical activity that is especially good for building cardiovascular fitness. The word *aerobic* means "with oxygen." In aerobic activities, your body supplies oxygen to keep you going. Active aerobic activity is continuous activity that makes your heart beat faster than normal to supply your body with the oxygen it needs. Examples of active aerobic activities are running, swimming, in-line skating, aerobic dance, and biking at vigorous intensity.

The word *active* is used in combination with the terms *aerobics, sports,* and *recreation* when describing activities at the second level of the pyramid. This is to make it clear that activities at the second level are vigorous. Moderate lifestyle activities at the first level of the pyramid are also considered to be aerobic because your body can supply enough oxygen to allow you to keep doing these activities for long periods of time. But they're not considered to be active aerobics because they're not vigorous enough to build optimal levels of cardiovascular fitness.

Active sports and **active recreation** also require the heart to beat faster and breathing to be faster than normal. When done for at least 20 minutes at a time at least three days a week, these activities build cardiovascular fitness and provide health benefits. Examples of active sports are tennis, basketball, badminton, volleyball, and soccer. Examples of active recreation are hiking, backpacking, and recreational games such as Ultimate.

Exercise is a word used to describe physical activity that is done especially to build physical fitness. The third level of the teen activity pyramid describes exercises that are designed to build muscle fitness and flexibility. Experts recommend that teens do **muscle fitness exercises** (such as push-ups and curl-ups) at least two days a week and **flexibility exercises** (such as stretching) at least three days a week. Muscle fitness exercises help you to build strong bones and prevent **muscle** injury. Flexibility exercises also help you prevent injury.

At the top of the teen pyramid is inactivity. The pyramid provides a small space for this level to encourage teens to limit periods of unproductive inactivity. Examples of unproductive inactivity include time spent performing "light" activities such as watching TV and playing computer games. Too much unproductive inactivity isn't good for your health or fitness. It can also limit your productivity in school and in performing other important daily tasks.

Inactivity as used in the pyramid doesn't include productive rest, such as sleep that allows recovery from the day's activities. For example, teens need at least nine hours of sleep each day. Teens also need time for relaxation and productive light activities, such as reading and doing homework.

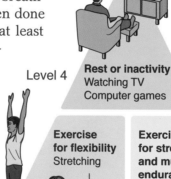
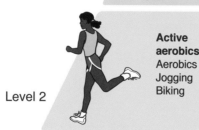
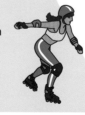
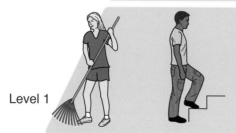
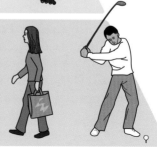

Level 4
Rest or inactivity
Watching TV
Computer games

Level 3
Exercise for flexibility
Stretching

Exercise for strength and muscular endurance
Resistance training
Calisthenics

Level 2
Active aerobics
Aerobics
Jogging
Biking

Active sports and recreation
Tennis
Basketball
In-line skating

Level 1
Lifestyle physical activity
Walk rather than ride
Climb the stairs
Do yard work
Play golf
Go bowling
Go fishing

The Physical Activity Pyramid for teens includes many types of activities.

Adapted, by permission, from C. Corbin and R. Lindsey, 2005, *Fitness for life*, 5th ed. (Champaign, IL: Human Kinetics), 64.

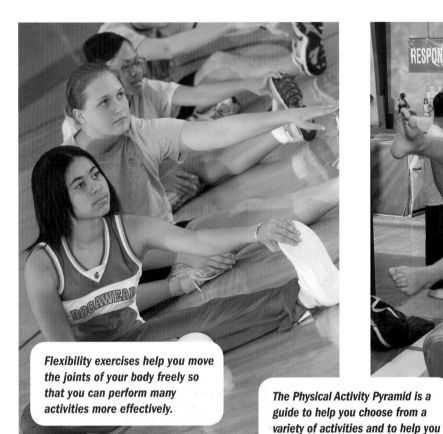

Fligibility exercises help you move the joints of your body freely so that you can perform many activities more effectively.

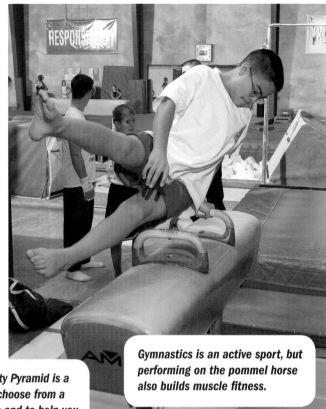

Gymnastics is an active sport, but performing on the pommel horse also builds muscle fitness.

The Physical Activity Pyramid is a guide to help you choose from a variety of activities and to help you determine the benefits of each. Depending on how you perform them, activities can be placed in different levels of the pyramid.

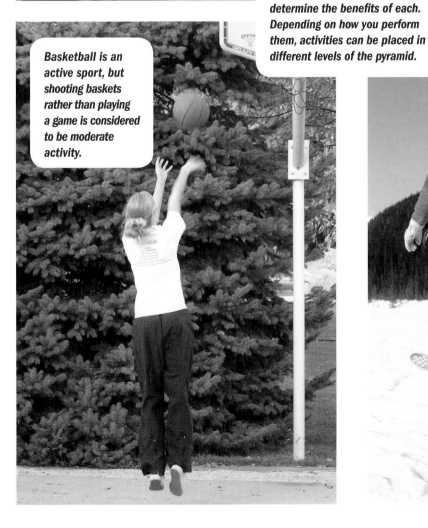

Basketball is an active sport, but shooting baskets rather than playing a game is considered to be moderate activity.

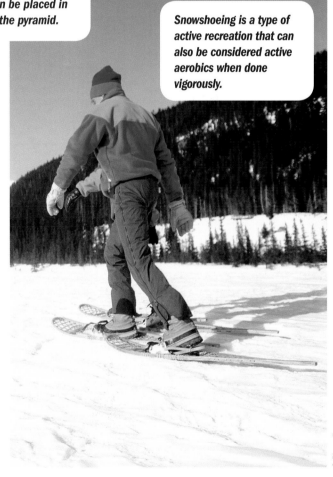

Snowshoeing is a type of active recreation that can also be considered active aerobics when done vigorously.

Why Do I Need Physical Activity?

Physical activities have many benefits. They help you to be healthy and to have good physical fitness. They can also help you look your best and enjoy yourself. Finding one or more physical activities that you enjoy helps you have fun and meet other people. Different kinds of physical activities have different benefits. Some of these benefits are described in later chapters of this book.

How Do I Start?

Before you start a physical activity such as playing a game or sport, it's best to warm up. The **warm-up** helps you to get your heart, blood vessels, muscles, and other body systems ready so that they'll work well and so that you won't injure your muscles. It's best to start with an activity such as slow jogging or fast walking. This part of the warm-up is called the "general warm-up" and gets the muscles warm. It's sometimes called the "heart warm-up" because it also gets the heart ready for activity.

Experts recommend that you start with a general warm-up and then perform stretching exercises to warm up the muscles in several areas of your body. The calf stretch and the side stretch are examples of stretching exercises that you might use in a warm-up. Your teacher will show you other warm-up exercises, and you will learn more about stretching exercises in chapter 6.

Click Student Info ▶ Topic 1.2

After your workout, it's best not to stop abruptly. Do some slow jogging or fast walking to help the heart and the rest of your body cool down. This type of **cool-down** causes the muscles of the legs to act as pumps and push blood back to the heart. If you stop vigorous exercise too quickly, blood can collect in your legs for a longer time, resulting in a slower recovery.

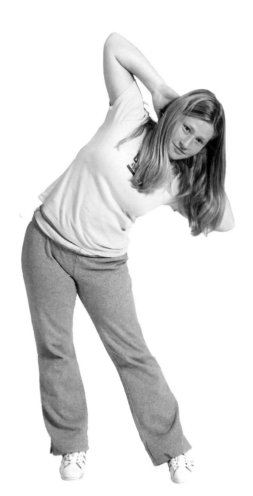

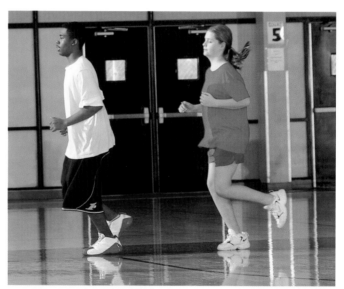

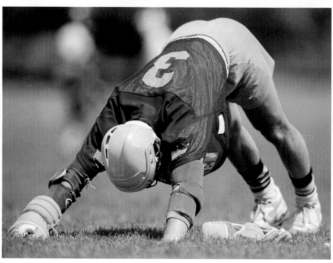

Walking or slow jogging can serve as a general warm-up or cool-down (above right). A warm-up or cool-down also includes stretching exercises (above and below right).

Moving Together: Communication

Do you ever feel as though you really click with certain people? When they say something, you know just what they mean? When you tell them something, they really understand what you're trying to say? Do you ever have times when plans get all messed up because you and your friends are not communicating?

Paulette just had a very bad day. When she got up in the morning, she realized she needed her clean workout clothes, and they were still rolled up in a ball in her gym bag. She was angry with herself for forgetting to wash them. When her mom asked her what was wrong, she snapped, "Never mind. It's not your problem." Then she felt bad about snapping at her mom.

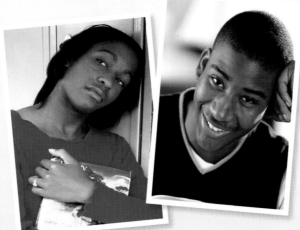

When she got to first period, she was horrified when Mr. Jasper asked her to submit the first draft of her English assignment. She was sure he had said it was due tomorrow.

At lunch, Donte asked her if she wanted to shoot hoops after school. She liked basketball, but she couldn't tell if he was asking her for real or just teasing her. Although Paulette thought it would be fun, she decided she didn't want to be embarrassed if he was just kidding. She decided to play it safe by not going.

That evening, Donte called Paulette at home. "I waited for you on the court," he said, sounding annoyed. "I thought you liked basketball."

Paulette felt sick to her stomach because Donte really *had* wanted her to play and she missed her chance. She felt bummed out for the rest of the night.

Discussion Questions

1. What else could Paulette have said to her mom?
2. What could Paulette do next time to make sure she understands the English teacher's expectations so that she isn't surprised by the deadline?
3. Why do you think Paulette wasn't sure if Donte was sincere about playing basketball?
4. What could Paulette do differently next time?
5. What could Donte do differently next time?

Click Student Info ▶ Topic 1.3

Guidelines for Effective Communication

Some strategies help us communicate better and avoid problems. You may do these already, but if you don't, you should give them a try.

▶ *Focus on one thing at a time.* It's hard to focus if you try to think about several things at once. Taking time to really focus on the person you are talking to helps your communication. Give your full attention when your teacher or friend is talking.

▶ *Write it down.* One reason for poor communication is that we sometimes forget what others have said. If the conversation is about something you have to do, or about an assignment, it's good to write it down. Using a planner or notebook is better than writing it on a random slip of paper that might be misplaced. Make it a habit to check your list several times each day.

▶ *Ask if you have questions.* When you're not sure if someone is kidding, it's usually best to ask. For example, you might say, "Are you kidding me, or do you really mean it?" This may clear things up quickly.

▶ *Get the person's attention.* When you really want to discuss something with someone, it helps to get the other person's attention before you start to share your information. "Hey, James, I wanted to ask you something." This kind of statement gets the person's attention and increases the chance that the person will pay attention to you.

▶ *Look at the person you are talking to.* When someone is talking to you, let that person know you're listening by looking at the person and nodding. Saying something back also helps. You might say, "If I heard you right, you said that you're interested in going to the movie, but just not on Saturday." Talking like this can feel strange at first, but it helps keep things straight.

▶ *Give your attention to others.* If you want others to pay attention to you, make sure you pay attention to them.

▶ *Take a minute to prepare.* In the late afternoon or early evening, take a minute to think about the next day and what you'll need for your activities. This will help you be more prepared. It also leaves enough time to ask someone else for help when you need it.

Activitygram

Activitygram is a computer program that helps you find out whether you get enough physical activity from each of the levels of the Physical Activity Pyramid for teens each day. Studies show that most teens become less active as they grow older and that many do not get enough activity for good health and fitness. Activitygram will show you whether you're among the teens who are active or inactive.

You can learn more about Activitygram at the *Fitness for Life: Middle School* Web site. The Activitygram shown at right is a sample report generated for a typical 13-year-old girl who measured her activity patterns for three days.

Click Student Info ▶ Topic 1.4

ACTIVITYGRAM®

Cooper, Jordan
Fall AG: 10/18/2006
Cityville Middle School
Cityville Middle School District

MINUTES OF ACTIVITY

Non-School Day
School Day 1
School Day 2
Goal — 60 Minutes

Minutes of Activity: 30, 60, 120

MESSAGES • MESSAGES • MESSAGES

The chart shows the number of minutes that you reported doing moderate (medium) or vigorous (hard) activity on each day. Congratulations, your log indicates that you are doing at least 60 minutes on some days. For optimal fitness and wellness perform at least 60 minutes each day. For fun and variety, try some new activities with family and friends on the weekends.

TIME PROFILE

Non-School Day
Vigorous / Moderate / Light / Rest
7AM 8 9 10 11 12 1 2 3 4 5 6 7 8 910PM

School Day 1
Vigorous / Moderate / Light / Rest
7AM 8 9 10 11 12 1 2 3 4 5 6 7 8 910PM

School Day 2
Vigorous / Moderate / Light / Rest
7AM 8 9 10 11 12 1 2 3 4 5 6 7 8 910PM

LEGEND:
◆ Most of the time (20 minutes)   ■ All of the time (30 minutes)
▲ Some of the time (10 minutes)   ☐ TV/Computer Time

The time profile shows the activity level you reported for each 30 minute period of the day. Your results show that you were not active during school but that you were active after school and on weekends. If it is not possible to be active during school in PE or recess try to be more active after school and on weekends. Keep up the good work!

ACTIVITY PROFILE

Rest
Muscular Activity / Flexibility Activity
Aerobic Sports / Aerobic Activity
Lifestyle Activity

Legend
☐ Participated in these types of activities
☐ Did not participate in these types of activities

The activity pyramid reveals the different types of activity that you reported doing over a few days. Your results indicate that you participated in regular lifestyle activity and some aerobic activity. This is great! Try to add some additional activity from the 3rd level of the pyramid.

Your results indicate that you spend an average of 2 hours per day watching TV or working on the computer. While some time on these activities is okay, you should try to limit the total time to less than 2 hours.

ACTIVITYGRAM provides information about your normal levels of physical activity. The ACTIVITYGRAM report shows what types of activity you do and how often you do them. It includes the information that you previously entered for two or three days during one week.

© 2005, 2006 The Cooper Institute

Take It Home

Friends and Family

"I didn't hear you."

"I heard you but I didn't know what you meant."

"Are you talking to me?"

Have you ever said any of these things? If you have, it means that you may be talking to someone else, but you're not communicating. Communication means giving *and* receiving information. So if information is given but not received, you're not really communicating.

Communicating with others happens all the time. Good communication helps people understand each other, and poor communication can cause us all sorts of problems. Maybe your mom didn't know you hate purple (perhaps because you never told her), and now she's given you something that you really dislike. You're both frustrated. Or maybe your friend seemed to criticize your new haircut and then say she was just kidding. You don't know what to think, and now you feel uptight.

Communicating with family and friends is important. Being active every day sometimes requires lots of support from people around you, and that requires good communication.

Maybe you need to ask someone for a ride to a game, or get your friends to agree on a time and place to meet. In most games, of course, you need to come to an agreement about the rules. To enjoy physical activity with family and friends, you need to know the kinds of activities they enjoy. All this takes lots of good communication.

Use the worksheet supplied by your teacher to talk to a friend or family member about the Physical Activity Pyramid. By asking questions and getting answers about activities you both like to perform, you're communicating. Use the results of your communications to plan some special physical activities, such as a family walk or a bike ride with friends.

Lesson Review

▶ What is physical activity?

▶ Why do you need physical activity?

▶ What is a warm-up, and why is it necessary?

▶ What are some guidelines for effective communication?

Introduction to Physical Fitness

Lesson Vocabulary

body composition, calipers, cardiovascular fitness, energy, Fitnessgram, flexibility, force, health-related fitness, healthy fitness zone, muscular endurance, physical fitness, sedentary, skill-related fitness, strength

Click Student Info ▶ Topic 1.5

Some people think that **physical fitness** is just one thing. Actually, there are many parts to physical fitness. Do you know about the different parts of fitness? Do you know how to tell whether you're physically fit? Do you know what energy, force, and movement are and how they help you to be efficient and effective in activity? When you finish this lesson, you'll know the answers to these questions.

What Is Physical Fitness?

One of the main reasons for performing the activities in the Physical Activity Pyramid is to build physical fitness. Teens who are active and fit feel good, look good, and are more likely to be healthy than are teens who are **sedentary,** or inactive. Physical fitness also helps you to perform well in sports and games, as well as in many jobs such as police officer, construction worker, archeologist, or photographer. So, what is physical fitness? How can you tell whether you have it?

The general definition of *physical fitness* is the ability of the body systems to work together efficiently. But physical fitness isn't just one thing; it is many things. Experts now agree that

there are at least 11 parts of physical fitness. Five of these parts make up **health-related fitness.** These parts are especially important because they help you to be healthy. The five parts of health-related physical fitness are cardiovascular fitness, strength, muscular endurance, flexibility, and body composition. In addition to making you healthy, the five parts of health-related fitness provide the other benefits described earlier.

- **Cardiovascular fitness** is the ability of the heart, lungs, blood vessels, and blood to work efficiently and to supply the body with oxygen. Cardiovascular fitness allows you to do physical activity for a long time without getting tired. Cardiovascular fitness is sometimes called aerobic capacity or cardiorespiratory fitness. Jogging, swimming, and biking for long periods of time require good cardiovascular fitness.
- **Strength** is the ability of muscles to lift a heavy weight or exert a lot of force. Weightlifters, parents or workers who lift children, and gymnasts must have good strength.
- **Muscular endurance** is the ability to use muscles for a long period of time without getting tired. You must have strength, but you also must be able to use your strength for an extended period. For example, doing a few push-ups is an indicator of strength, but doing many push-ups is a measure of endurance. Hiking and backpacking are other activities that require muscular endurance. Professional movers require muscular endurance to load and unload household belongings.
- **Flexibility** is the ability to move all body parts and joints freely. Flexibility requires long muscles that allow your joints to move as they should. Dancers, cheerleaders, and football kickers need good flexibility.
- **Body composition** is the combination of all tissues that make up the body such as bones, muscles, organs, and body fat. Bones, muscles, and organs are called lean body tissue. Most of your body should consist of lean tissue rather than fat. You can use an instrument known as **calipers** to measure the fat under your skin to determine your body fat level.

Click Student Info ▶ Topic 1.6

You need all five parts of health-related fitness.

In addition to the five parts of health-related physical fitness, there are six parts that are called **skill-related fitness.** These parts of physical fitness don't relate directly to your health, but they do help you to perform well in sports and physical activity. You'll learn more about skill-related physical fitness in chapter 2.

five parts of health-related fitness, you'll need to do at least five different tests to see if you have good health-related fitness. **Fitnessgram** is a national fitness test that includes tests for all parts of health-related physical fitness. You'll learn more about the tests later in this book.

Click Student Info ▶ Topic 1.7

How Do I Know if I'm Physically Fit?

Experts have developed many tests that you can use to see if you're physically fit. Because there are

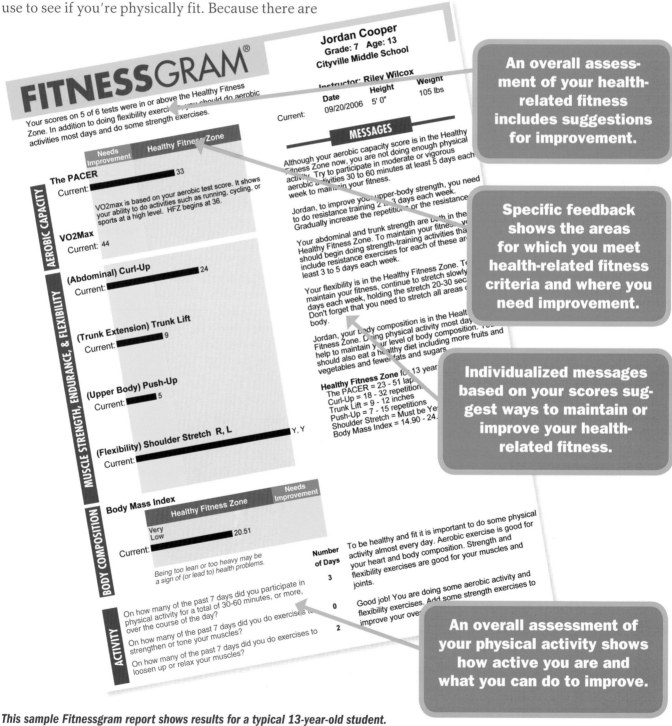

This sample Fitnessgram report shows results for a typical 13-year-old student.

Adapted, by permission, from The Cooper Institute, 2005, *Fitnessgram/Activitygram test administration manual, updated 4th ed.* (Champaign, IL: Human Kinetics).

Biomechanical Principles:
Energy, Force, and Movement

Energy and force are necessary for producing human movement.

Energy means "available power." We use electric power to provide energy to light our houses and to power appliances such as television sets and washing machines. Electric companies provide the energy using coal, gas, oil, wind, solar, or nuclear sources. The food you eat provides the energy that allows your muscles to contract. When your muscles contract, they produce **force** that causes the bones to move, creating movement of body parts and total body movement. For example, when the muscles of your legs contract, your legs move. Leg movement allows you to move the whole body, such as when you walk.

You move most efficiently when the force produced by the muscles is applied in the direction in which you want to move. For example, when you throw a ball, it's best to apply force to the ball by moving your arm in the direction you want the ball to go. The more force the muscles apply, the farther the ball will travel. Also, the longer the force is applied, the more force you can apply. If you reach back a long way before throwing the ball, you can apply force forward for a longer time, and you can throw the ball farther. When you walk or run and do other movements, the same rules apply.

Sir Isaac Newton is credited with developing three laws of motion. These laws are related to force and how it's used to create and regulate motion. Much of the information provided here is based on Newton's laws. For more information about force and Newton's laws relating to force, visit the *Fitness for Life: Middle School* Web site.

Click Student Info ▶ Topic 1.8

- ▶ Point your feet and toes straight ahead (see photo below left), not to the side (see photo below right). This allows the force from your legs and feet to keep you moving forward and doesn't waste force to one side or the other.
- ▶ Swing your arms in line with the direction of the intended movement to avoid wasting force. Swinging your arms to the side reduces the forward force that you can produce with your legs.
- ▶ Avoid twisting your body. Keep your trunk (hips, belly, and chest) facing the direction you are walking or running.
- ▶ Apply force for the full time that your foot is on the ground. When you are in the air (such as in running) no force can be applied and so you can't increase your speed.
- ▶ To move faster, apply more force. Fast walking and running will require you to apply more force than slow walking.

Principle in Practice

Correct application of force is important for efficient and effective movement in normal daily activities and in physical activities of all kinds. Work with a partner to see if you're applying force properly when walking and running. Have your partner watch your arms and legs to see whether your movements are straight ahead or to the sides. If your movements include motion to the sides, try to change the way you walk or run to be more efficient.

Applying the Principle

To move well, you need to know how to use force efficiently and effectively. In walking and running, for example, it's best to apply the force in line with the direction of movement. Experts have discovered several rules that will help you use the force that your legs produce when pushing off the ground.

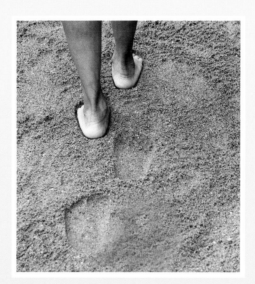

Good force application.

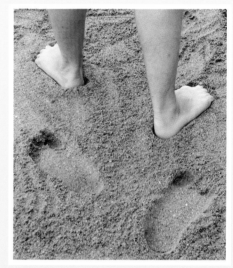

Inefficient force application.

What Else Affects My Physical Fitness?

As you learned in the first lesson of this chapter, the best way to build physical fitness is to do regular physical activity. Being active will help you to build all parts of health-related fitness.

But some people will have an easier time than others in getting fit. Scientists have shown that among young people, heredity is very important to fitness. In other words, some people may score better on fitness tests than others because of bodily characteristics that they inherit. Older people in the class who have grown taller and stronger may perform better on tests of strength but may score lower in other areas such as flexibility.

For all of these reasons, you shouldn't compare your fitness scores with other people. Improving and getting in the healthy fitness zone are the most important concerns.

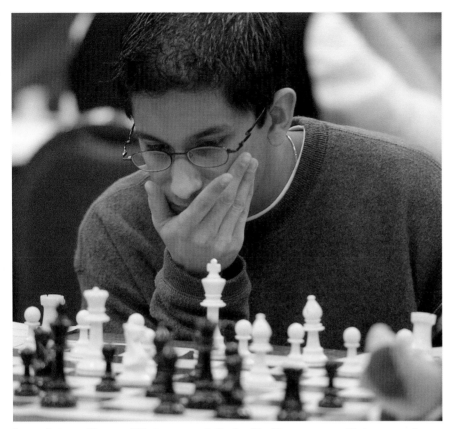

Improving your fitness will help you reach the healthy fitness zone and help you perform well in all kinds of activities, including those that require long periods of concentration.

When you have completed each of the Fitness-gram tests, you can rate your fitness. To have good health-related fitness, you should be in the **healthy fitness zone** for each of the five parts of health-related fitness. If you're below the healthy fitness zone, you're in the low fitness zone, and you should consider taking steps to improve your fitness. You can be low in one part of fitness and in the healthy fitness zone for other parts of fitness.

Once you achieve the healthy fitness zone for a fitness part, try to improve your fitness within the zone. This will help you perform well in sports, games, and active jobs, and it will help you feel and look your best. Although we encourage you to be in the healthy fitness zone, exceptionally high levels of fitness aren't necessary for good health. Once you're in the "zone," you can decide how much additional fitness you need to reach your personal goals.

FIT FACT

Children are the most active group of people, followed by teens, adults, and senior citizens. The same is true for most animals— think of bear cubs, puppies, or kittens playing while the parents watch.

Lesson Review

▶ What is physical fitness?

▶ How do you know if you're physically fit?

▶ How are energy and force important to performing physical activities?

▶ Do things other than physical activity affect your physical fitness?

Chapter Review

Number your paper from 1 to 5. Read each question. After the number for the question, write a word or a phrase that best answers the question. The page number where you can find the answer is listed after the question.

1. What do you call the type of physical activity in the first level of the Physical Activity Pyramid? (page 3)
2. What word describes physical activity for which the body can supply enough oxygen to keep doing the activity for long periods? (page 4)
3. What is the name of the computer program that can determine if teens get enough physical activity? (page 8)
4. What word describes the ability of your muscles to lift a weight or exert force? (page 9)
5. What phrase describes having enough fitness for good health? (page 12)

Number your paper from 6 to 10. Next to each number, write the letter of the best answer.

6. exercise	**a.** a group of health-related fitness tests
7. flexibility	**b.** use of energy to cause movement
8. Fitnessgram	**c.** physical activity done for fitness
9. force	**d.** using body systems efficiently
10. physical fitness	**e.** good range of motion

Number your paper from 11 to 15. Follow the directions to answer each question or statement.

11. Draw a picture of the Physical Activity Pyramid and include labels for each of the activities included in it.
12. Give examples of guidelines for communicating effectively.
13. Describe some exercises that are good to include in a warm-up.
14. Explain the difference between moderate physical activity and vigorous physical activity.
15. Describe the five parts of health-related physical fitness and give examples of each.

Ask the Authors

I'm on a sports team and do several hours of sports each day. Do I have to do lifestyle activities to meet the teen activity recommendation?

Get the answer and ask your own questions at the *Fitness for Life: Middle School* Web site.

Click Student Info ▶ Topic 1.9

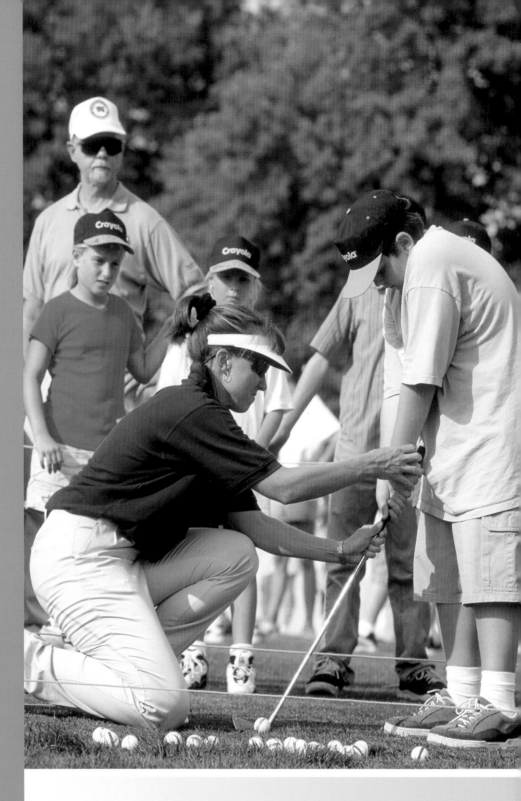

2

Learning Skills for Enjoying Physical Activity

Learning Motor Skills

Lesson Vocabulary

agility, balance, coordination, motor skills, motor units, performance skills, power, practice, reaction time, skill, skill-related fitness, speed, sport skills

▶ www.fitnessforlife.org/middleschool/
Click Student Info ▶ Topic 2.1

Do you know the difference between skills and skill-related fitness? Do you know why you need skills and skill-related fitness? When you finish this lesson, you'll know the answers to these questions. You'll also know more about participating in groups, both as a leader and as a member.

What Are Skills?

In chapter 1 you learned that health-related physical fitness helps you to be healthy, to feel and look good, and to enjoy life. Having good health-related physical fitness also helps you to perform well in sports, in most jobs, and even when doing schoolwork because you're better able to resist fatigue and stay focused on your work. Although health-related physical fitness is important to performing well, it's only one of several important factors that help you perform your best.

Two other important factors in helping you to be a good performer are skills and **skill-related fitness. Skill** is your ability to do a specific task, such as dribbling a basketball or performing a dance step. Performing a skill involves using your muscles and nerves together with your brain. You learned some very basic skills early in life, including crawling, walking, running, skipping, and jumping. When you perform a skill, your brain signals your nerves, and your nerves stimulate your muscles and tell them how to move. At first a specific skill may be hard to do, but after a lot of practice, the brain, muscles, and nerves learn to work together so that your movements become almost automatic.

You probably won't remember it, but walking is a skill that was hard for you when you first tried it. You may remember learning to ride a bike. It's also a skill that was hard at first. But you kept trying it over and over again until you got good at it. Both walking and riding a bike are specific tasks that require practice. As you try different types of physical activities, you'll need to learn different skills including those used in light, moderate, and vigorous activities. Examples of skills used in light activity are typing, playing a musical instrument, and playing a computer game. Skills used in moderate activity include using tools for digging or raking when working in the yard.

You have to learn many skills when performing vigorous activities such as sports. These skills are sometimes called **sport skills** because they're necessary for you to be good at sports and games. Like walking, running, and jumping, sport skills are learned with practice. Each sport and game has many skills, so you'll have to practice different skills for different sports. For example, kicking isn't a part of softball or baseball, and batting isn't used in soccer. But many sport skills are common to several sports. Serving in tennis is similar to overhand serving in volleyball, but in volleyball you don't use a racket. The tennis serve motion is also similar to an overhand pitch in baseball or a quarterback's throw in football. Skills you learn for one sport can also be used to help you perform another.

Sometimes names other than *sport skills* are used. One example is **motor skills.** We often think of a motor as being the same as a car's engine. In this case *motor* means something else. Nerves and muscles that work together when signaled by the brain are called **motor units.** These units work together to cause body parts such as the fingers, arms, and legs to move when you want them to. Because skills are used in activities other than sports, they're sometimes

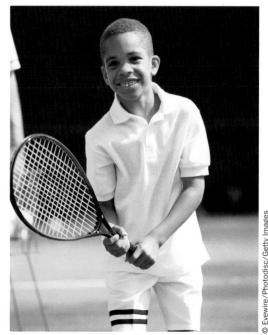

Different sports require different skills.

© Eyewire/Photodisc/Getty Images

referred to as **performance skills.** Whether we call them skills, motor skills, sport skills, or performance skills, we all need to be able to perform them. We all need to be able to use our brains, our nerves, and our muscles to cause our bodies to move and do our daily activities. With **practice** we learn these skills and are able to function effectively.

With practice anyone can learn skills. However, the younger you are, the easier you may learn skills. We know that most basic skills and sport skills are learned in elementary and middle school. That's why teachers and parents encourage young people to learn skills early. People who learn skills early in life are more likely to be active for a lifetime than are people who don't learn skills early.

What Is Skill-Related Fitness?

Now that you've learned about skills, it's important that you learn about skill-related fitness. Skill-related fitness refers to abilities that help people learn skills. The six parts of skill-related fitness—agility, balance, coordination, power, reaction time, and speed—are described in table 2.1. Skill-related fitness isn't the same as skill. Having good skill-related fitness does help you to learn skills. For example, balance is important in many activities. If you have good balance, you'll be able to learn specific skills, such as in-line skating, more easily than if balance is hard for you. Different people have different skill-related fitness abilities based on their heredity, their

age, and the amount of experience they've had in a variety of physical activities. But balance practice can improve your general balance, just as skill practice can improve your performance of specific skills. Most people are good in a few parts of skill-related fitness and not so good in others. Later, you'll get a chance to assess your skill-related fitness. For now, look over the photos and descriptions of the parts of skill-related fitness on page 17. Think about activities you do that require different parts of skill-related fitness.

Click Student Info ▶ Topic 2.2

Why Do I Need Motor Skills and Skill-Related Fitness?

There are many goals designed to help all of us to become healthy people. A major health goal is regular physical activity among all people, especially young people who are still in school. We know that adults aren't as active as young people and that elementary school and middle school students are more active than high school students. So finding a way to help young people stay active as they get older is an important health goal. Learning skills can help you to enjoy activities that you can use to stay active now and later in life.

Click Student Info ▶ Topic 2.3

Most experts agree that learning specific skills and having good skill-related fitness are both important. But skill-related fitness is based on factors that aren't always in your control, so there's a limit to how much you can improve it. There are drills you can do to help, but you shouldn't be discouraged if it's hard for you to improve on some parts of skill-related fitness. Also, not all people will be able to develop skills equally. Some people learn skills faster than others, but with good practice all people can learn skills well enough to enjoy most physical activities.

You may want to do some self-tests (also called self-assessments) to learn about your skill-related fitness. Knowing about your skill-related fitness can help you decide which skills will be easiest for you to learn.

Balance is required for performing a wide variety of motor skills.

Table 2.1

Parts of Skill-Related Physical Fitness

Agility is the ability to change body positions quickly and keep your body under control when it is moving. Agility helps you in activities such as rope games, dancing, wrestling, and defending in football and basketball.

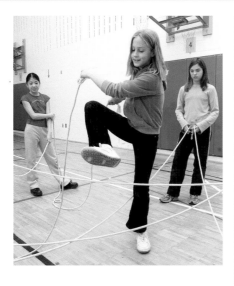

Power is the ability to combine strength with speed while moving. A shot putter combines strength with speed to perform with power. A softball player who swings the bat quickly and with a lot of force demonstrates power.

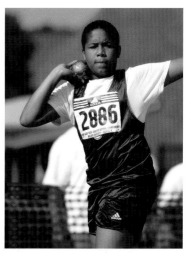

Balance is the ability to keep your body in a steady position while standing or moving. Balance helps you to ride a surfboard, ride a bike, and do activities such as the balance beam in gymnastics.

Reaction time is the ability to move quickly when you get a signal to start moving. A swimmer or runner starting a race needs good reaction time.

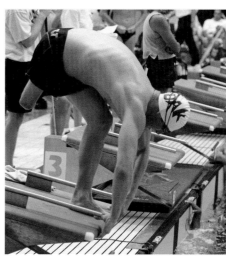

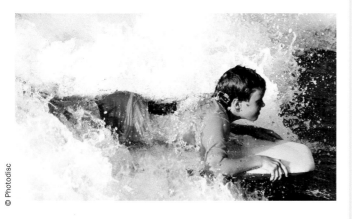

© Photodisc

Coordination is the ability of body parts to work together when you perform an activity. Hitting a ball requires the use of your eyes together with your hands and arms. Jumping hurdles, kickboxing, and aerobic dance require your eyes, feet, and legs. Kicking and performing dance steps require coordination.

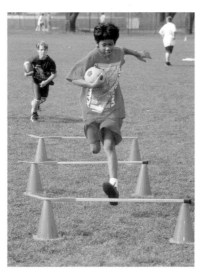

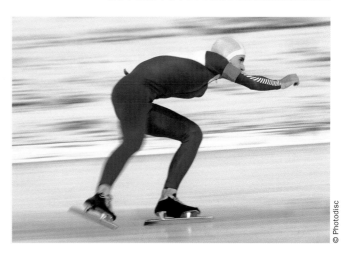

© Photodisc

Speed is the ability to get from one place to another in the shortest possible time. You can have speed of your whole body, such as when you skate or run fast, or speed of body parts, such as when you move your hands very quickly to steal a ball from another person in a basketball game.

Moving Together: Full Participation

Can you remember a time when you were the leader of a group in a physical activity setting? How did you perform as a leader? Were you successful at getting all members of your group to participate? What strategies did you use to promote participation? How do you feel when people don't pay attention to you? How do you feel when some members of a group do less work than others?

Jimmy and Molly were in physical education class. The class was doing an exercise routine that required them to try several different skills and then do them to music. They were assigned to a group to read about a skill and then show the class how to do it properly. Molly was the group leader. She read the directions for the skill, showed the group a picture of it, and asked all group members to try it.

When it was her group's turn, Molly was going to read the class a description of the skill and have all group members demonstrate at the same time. But some group members didn't pay attention. Two group members were talking about other things. Jimmy just quietly stood to the side.

Discussion Questions

1. What could Molly do to get all group members to participate in the activity?
2. How could Jimmy help Molly to keep the group working together?
3. What other suggestions do you have to help the group complete its assignment?
4. Are there any other questions we should ask?

Guidelines for Full Participation

Everybody learns faster and better when all members of a group are actively involved in the group activity. Two kinds of guidelines can help the group to have full participation: group leader guidelines and group member guidelines.

If you're the leader of a group, follow these guidelines.

▶ *Use basic leadership skills.* These include things such as speaking with a strong voice, maintaining eye contact when you talk to other group members, and showing enthusiasm for what you're doing.

▶ *Ask questions of the group members.* By asking questions of others in the group, you increase the participation by all group members.

▶ *Ask group members to help demonstrate skills.* You can show your enthusiasm by demonstrating some of the skills yourself, but you can also involve others in the group by asking them to demonstrate skills.

▶ *Have all group members practice the skill together.* If group members practice the skill with you, they may feel more involved in the group's activity.

▶ *Give positive feedback to those who try.* Thank them for their effort.

▶ *Tell group members that it is OK to make a mistake.* We all make mistakes at first. Practice will help everyone improve.

If you're asked to participate as a member of a group, follow these guidelines.

▶ *Help the leader by participating.* In this class all students will get a chance to be a group leader. When you're the leader, you'll want the help of other students, so giving your help when you're a group member will help get the cooperation of others when you're the leader.

▶ *Avoid talking when the leader is talking.* This is one of the best ways to help the leader. Also, paying close attention to the leader will help you learn the skill the leader is teaching.

▶ *Give your best effort in all activities.* Effort is one of the most important factors in learning. Most people don't succeed the first time. If you get in the habit of working at something, you'll find that you can do all sorts of things that you thought were hard at first.

Click Student Info ▶ Topic 2.4

Consider these examples when choosing activities. If you have good balance, you may decide that gymnastics is a good choice. If you have good coordination, you may decide that tennis or baseball is a good choice. But your skill-related fitness shouldn't keep you from choosing an activity that you think you'll enjoy. The key is practicing the skills of the activity that you choose. With good practice and good instruction, any activity choice is a good one.

Click Student Info ▶ Topic 2.5

Enjoyment is a very good reason for learning skills. If you practice motor skills, you get better at performing them. The better you are, the more you enjoy the activity. And the more you enjoy the activity, the more you'll do it. Of course, many movement skills are important to daily living, too. Some skills help you to do important activities that don't build fitness and health. For example, you need to be able to write to do schoolwork, but writing isn't a movement skill that leads to fitness.

Once you have learned a skill, you need to keep practicing it as you grow older. The body of a teenager often changes rapidly. As you grow taller and

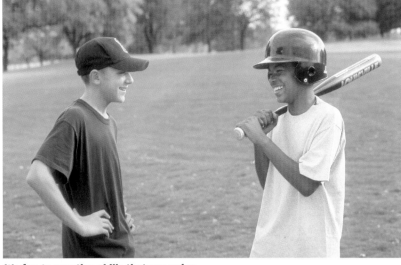

It's fun to practice skills that you enjoy.

your arms and legs grow longer, practice will help you adjust your performances to your new body size. As you grow bigger, practice will help you to move your body with greater speed and accuracy. These are both important in performing well in sports and other physical activities. As you grow, you'll also be able to apply more force with your body's longer levers (your arms and legs), allowing you to kick or throw a ball a greater distance.

Take It Home

Your Support Team

In NASCAR auto racing, drivers have support teams that help them in training and getting through the race. When drivers need fuel or their tires changed, they pull into the pit area and their team goes to work to get them ready to roll again. Wouldn't it be great if we each had a support team like that? Being on the support team of others and building support teams for ourselves are some of the most important things we do in life. Family, friends, teachers, and teammates may all be part of our support team.

Sometimes when we're feeling bad, we think that no one is on our team. Most people feel that way at one time or another, but if you think about it, you'll realize that you have quite a few people on your support team. Everyone has a different combination of people who are available to listen, share experiences, offer advice, and generally just help us through life. Some kids have one parent, some have two parents, and some have three or more. Some kids have grandparents, guardians, aunts, or uncles who are important in their lives. Some kids have brothers, sisters, nieces, or nephews that are best buddies. Neighbors, church members, teachers, coaches, recreation workers, and librarians can all be part of our support teams. A few

people is all it takes to make a real difference. Often we don't know how many people we have on our team until we run into a problem. Knowing who is on your team will help you identify people to help with your assignments in this class.

Use the worksheet supplied by your teacher to list people who are on your support team or who could be recruited to join your team. Then choose team members who can support your physical activity or practice with you this week. You can support and encourage their physical activity, too.

Click Student Info ▶ Topic 2.6

Lesson Review

▶ What are skills?

▶ What are the parts of skill-related fitness?

▶ Why are skills and skill-related fitness important?

▶ How can you encourage others to participate in a group that you're leading?

▶ How can you participate in a group that you're not leading?

The Importance of Practice

Lesson Vocabulary

feedback, first-class levers, lever, mental practice, paralysis by analysis, practice, routine, second-class levers, third-class levers

Click Student Info ▶ Topic 2.7

What is **practice,** and why should you do it? Do you know the best way to practice? When you finish this lesson, you'll know the answer to these ques-

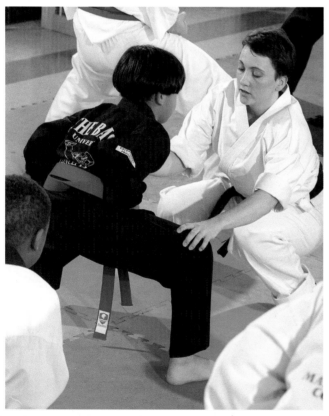

Perfect practice makes perfect.

tions. You'll also know more about how the levers of the body are used to help you to be active and perform skills.

What Is Practice, and Why Should I Do It?

Practice means repeating an action over and over to improve skill. One famous saying is "Practice makes perfect." This means that the more you practice a skill, the better you get at performing it. Practice can improve all kinds of skills, from daily performance skills such as brushing your teeth and typing on a computer to sport skills such as hitting, catching, and kicking. If you want to get better at a skill, the best thing you can do is practice it. But some kinds of practice are better than other kinds. For the best results, you should practice in the best possible way.

What Is the Best Way to Practice?

Not all practice is good practice. Some experts have changed the old saying to "Perfect practice makes perfect." They did this to let you know that there's a right way and a wrong way to practice skills. If you practice the wrong way, your performance won't get better; it may even get worse. So before you begin to practice a skill, be sure to get good instruction. Instruction from an expert such as your physical education teacher can help you to get the most from your practice.

Click Student Info ▶ Topic 2.8

Once you have chosen a skill that you want to learn, an instructor can show you how to perform it correctly and how to practice it in the best possible way. If you're doing a skill incorrectly and practice it incorrectly, you won't get better at performing the skill. A qualified instructor helps you by giving you **feedback.** Feedback is information that the instructor "feeds" or gives "back" to you after you perform a movement so you have a better idea of what you did. Feedback helps you to make appropriate changes so that you improve your performance. It's hard to tell when you're doing a skill correctly because you can't see yourself move. But an instructor can see your movements and help you make adjustments.

Biomechanical Principles: Levers

The levers of the body allow you to apply force to create movements of many different kinds.

A **lever** is a very basic machine. It is a bar or stiff, straight object that can be used to lift weight, increase force, or create speed. The bones of your body are levers that allow you to perform many skills. For example, the bones of your foot act as a lever when you push with your foot while you walk and run. The calf muscles shorten, causing your foot to push down against the ground. To do its work, a lever must have a pivot point at the middle or at the end of the lever.

When you use the foot as a lever in walking and running, the ankle is the pivot point and the bones of the foot are the levers. When you use the bones as levers in this way, they are called **first-class levers.** First-class levers can allow you to lift a heavy weight with a small amount of force. For example, first-class levers allow you to lift your whole body weight with the relatively small leg

muscles (see below). A first-class lever also causes a change in the direction of the force so that the muscles in the back of your lower leg, which pull upward on the back of your foot (your heel), make the front of your foot (your toes) push downward against the ground.

In a first-class lever, the fulcrum (or pivot point) is between the resistance (or weight) and the effort (or force). First-class levers can be used to either increase the force applied or increase the speed and distance of movement.

Second-class levers are not common in the body. However, a good example of a second class lever is a person doing a push-up (see below). The body is straight from the shoulders to the feet. It acts as a lever with the pivot at the feet. The weight of the body is near the center, near the waist, and the arms work at the shoulders to lift the body. The force required for the arms to lift the body is about half the total body weight.

First-class lever: Toe raise

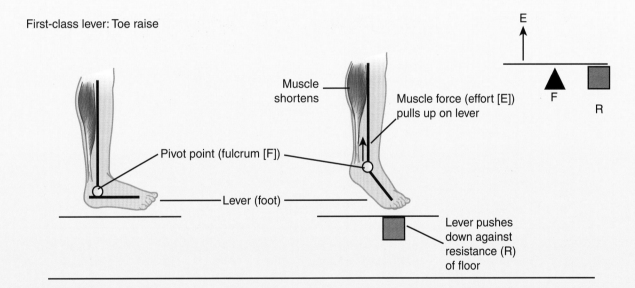

Second-class lever: Push-up

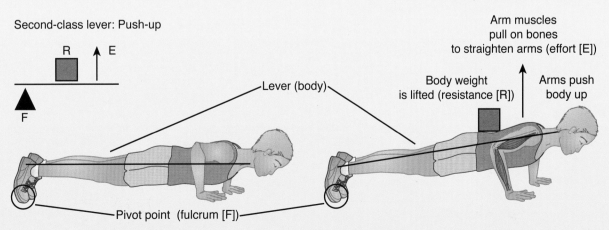

Click Student Info ▶ Topic 2.9

(continued)

Biomechanical Principles: Levers (continued)

In a second-class lever, the weight (or resistance) is between the fulcrum (or pivot point) and the effort (or force). Second class levers increase the force applied.

The most common type of levers in the body are **third-class levers**. In the human body, third-class levers have the pivot point at one end. The muscles apply force to the lever near the pivot. This causes the levers (your bones) to move. For example, in performing a biceps curl as illustrated below, the force of the contraction of the muscles of the upper arm pulls the lever (the lower arm) upward. The fulcrum or pivot point is the elbow, and the weight or resistance is the weight of the lower arm and the weight that's held in the hand. Third-class levers allow you to do fast movements such as throwing, kicking, or swinging a tennis racket. When you kick a ball, you use the bones of the upper leg, the lower leg, and the foot as third-class levers. For example, in kicking, the muscles of the hip move the upper leg forward, the muscles of the front of the upper leg move the lower leg forward, and the muscles of the lower leg move the foot forward and upward with great speed. That allows you to kick the ball a good distance if you make good contact with the ball when you kick it. Adding the levers one at a time results in even faster movement of the leg.

The levers of the arm work in a similar way when you swing an object such as a tennis racket or perform an exercise such as a biceps curl (see below). With practice, you can learn to move the levers with improved accuracy as well as improved speed.

In a third-class lever, the effort (or force applied) is between the weight (or resistance) and the fulcrum (or pivot point). Third-class levers increase speed.

You have to learn to use the levers of the body efficiently if you are going to learn a wide variety of skills. The more you practice, the better you become at using the body levers. With practice your timing improves so that you can kick, throw, jump, and do other skills faster and better. Practice helps your body memorize movements so that you can control them better and so that you can perform skills more accurately.

Applying the Principle

When you move one of the body's third-class levers such as the arm, the muscles move only a short distance but the end of the lever (the arm) moves a much greater distance. This creates a fast movement at the end of the lever (arm). This speed allows a person to throw a ball a great distance.

Put your hand on the muscles that are moving levers (bones) when you perform the following activities. Remember that the muscle causing the movement often is found closer to the center of the body than the moving part and does not attach near the fast-moving end of the bone, but closer to the other end of the lever.

▶ Kicking a hacky sack behind your back with your foot uses the muscles of the back of the upper leg and causes a backward movement of the lower leg (see *a* on page 23).

▶ Performing a forehand serve in badminton uses the muscles on the front of your shoulder and upper arm and causes a fast movement of the lower arm and the racket (see *b* on page 23).

▶ Performing a biceps curl using an elastic band uses the muscles on the front of your upper arm and causes movement of the lower arm (see *c* on page 23).

Notice that in each case, the end of the lever is moving farther and faster than the part closer to the pivot where the working muscle is attached.

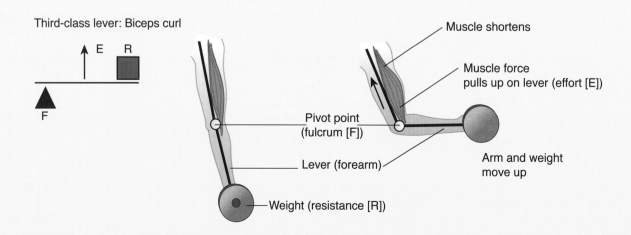

Third-class lever: Biceps curl

E   R

F

Muscle shortens

Muscle force pulls up on lever (effort [E])

Pivot point (fulcrum [F])

Lever (forearm)

Arm and weight move up

Weight (resistance [R])

In addition, other muscles and levers are involved in each of the motions described on the previous page. For example:

- Kicking a hacky sack with the back of your foot involves the muscles of the upper leg and lower leg and the levers of the lower leg and foot.
- Serving a birdie in badminton involves the muscles of the upper arm and forearm and the levers of the upper arm, forearm, and hand.
- Performing biceps curls against an elastic band involves the muscles of the upper arm and the forearm muscles that control the fingers.

Only some of the levers and muscles involved are described in the examples.

Principle in Practice

Using the body's levers helps you to perform skills that require speed. Practice kicking a ball using the levers of your leg. Start by kicking a ball that is lying on the ground. Think about using the levers in your upper and lower leg. The upper leg should move forward first, and then the lower leg. This will help you learn to use the same levers in punting a ball, such as in playing goalie in soccer. As you improve, the speed of your foot should increase and the distance you can kick will increase. Practice will also help you improve accuracy of kicking and throwing. However, it is best not to focus too much on accuracy when you are first learning. Once you have learned a skill properly (such as throwing or kicking), additional practice will help you improve accuracy. Practice using the levers of the arms in throwing a baseball or serving a volleyball. Use the worksheet provided by your teacher to investigate levers that you use every day.

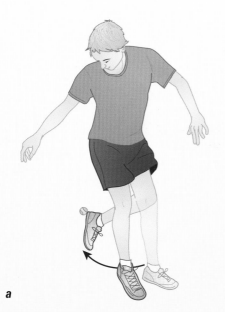

a

Using the legs as third-class levers.

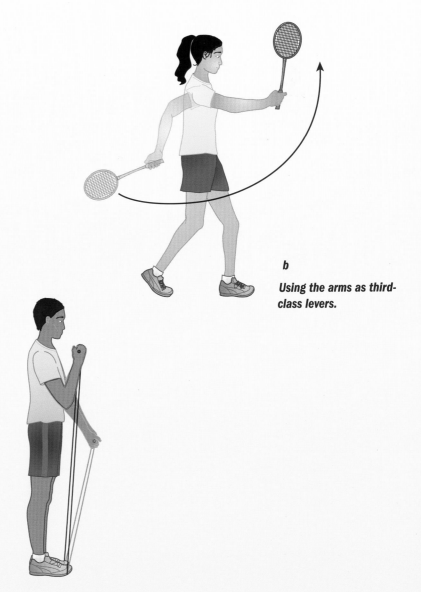

b

Using the arms as third-class levers.

c

Using the arms as third-class levers.

Scientists have found that the same neurons in your brain fire whether you're thinking about a movement or actually doing it.

A teacher is giving you feedback to help you improve your practice when he or she tells you if you're gripping the tennis racket properly or if you need to reach farther back when you swing the racket. Good feedback from an instructor helps you to practice better. A friend or family member can also provide feedback if the person knows what to look for when you practice. Some sport teams use video to get feedback to improve practice. If video is available to you, you could do the same.

Click Student Info ▶ Topic 2.10

Sometimes getting too much feedback when you're practicing can be a problem. Imagine practicing a skill such as the overhand volleyball serve. A friend is trying to help you. First, your friend says to toss the ball higher before hitting it. Then your friend says to toss the ball farther in front of you before hitting it. Then the advice is to jump before hitting the ball. Finally, you're told to keep your eye on the ball. This is just too much information for you to take in at one time. Too much information given at one time can lead to **paralysis by analysis**. Paralysis by analysis occurs when you have so much information (feedback) that you can't keep your focus—you're paralyzed by having too much to think about. Practice is best when you focus on one or two things at a time. Trying to think about too many things at once causes problems.

Mental practice can also help you to improve your skills. Mental practice is imagining performing a skill properly. Just thinking about performing the skill the right way can make your regular practice better. Mental practice can also help you develop a **routine** for doing the skill the same way every time. A routine is a series of steps that you go through

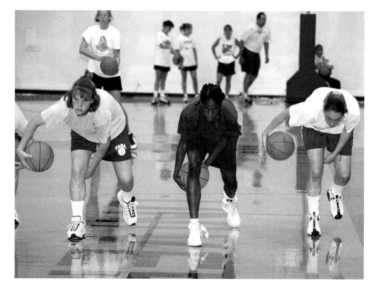

Practicing skills with friends helps keep practice interesting.

every time you perform a skill. For example, good putters in golf use the same routine each time they putt. Using a routine can improve your performance because you repeat the task over and over again in exactly the same way.

How Often Should I Practice?

Practice works best when you enjoy it and can focus on it. If you practice too long and get tired or bored, the practice is less effective because you're more likely to practice the movement incorrectly. That's why sport teams practice one skill for a while and then practice another. Finding ways to make practice fun, such as practicing with friends or using enjoyable practice drills, helps to keep it interesting and keep you focused. Although a practice session can be as long as a couple of hours, time spent practicing one skill may last only 5 to 30 minutes. Athletes often practice longer than this, but for most people longer practice sessions aren't necessary and may not be possible.

Practicing regularly is also important. If possible, daily practice is best. If you have limited time to practice, though, it's best to distribute practice over several days rather than do it for several hours on one day. In the same way that you forget facts that you learn, if you don't practice, your body "forgets" the best way to perform skills.

Lesson Review

▶ What is practice, and why should you do it?

▶ What are the important elements of good practice?

▶ How do body levers help you to perform physical activities?

▶ How often should you practice?

Chapter Review

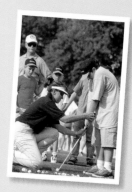

Number your paper from 1 to 5. Read each question. After the number for the question, write a word or a phrase that best answers the question. The page number where you can find the answer is listed after the question.

1. What word (or words) in this chapter describe(s) the ability to perform a specific task? (page 15)
2. What word describes nerves and muscles that work as a unit with the brain? (page 15)
3. What do you call the part of skill-related fitness that refers to the ability to change body positions quickly? (page 17)
4. What word describes the information you get from a teacher or from practice that helps you to change performance? (page 20)
5. What is the name of a basic machine described in this chapter? (page 21)

Number your paper from 6 to 10. Next to each number, write the letter of the best answer.

6. balance
7. practice
8. routine
9. paralysis by analysis
10. power

a. a combination of strength and speed
b. repeating a skill to improve performance
c. a series of steps for doing a skill the same way
d. ability to keep your body in a steady position
e. too much feedback that hurts performance

Number your paper from 11 to 15. Follow the directions to answer each question or statement.

11. Give examples of skills used in playing sports.
12. Explain the difference between skills and skill-related fitness.
13. Give examples of guidelines that help leaders get full participation from a group.
14. Describe the six parts of skill-related fitness and give examples of each.
15. Give examples of how the body's levers are used in physical activities.

Ask the Authors

Is it possible to get too much practice?
   Get the answer and ask your own questions at the *Fitness for Life: Middle School* Web site.

Click Student Info ▶ Topic 2.11

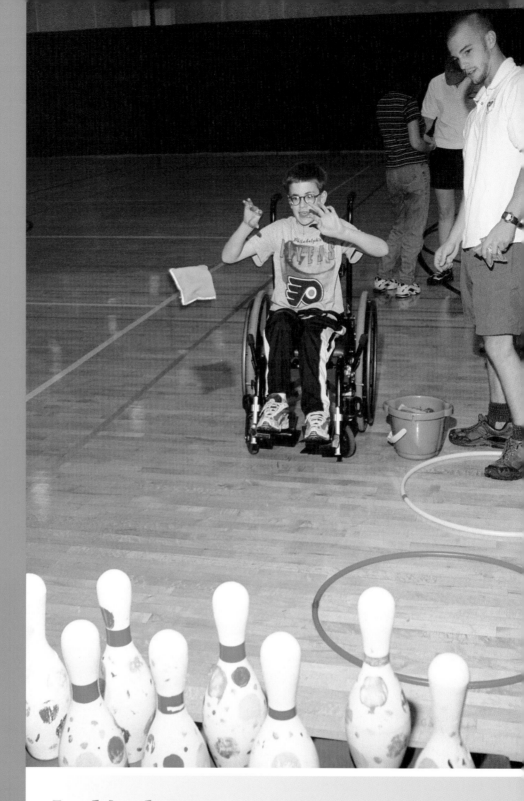

3

Lifestyle Physical Activity

Lifestyle Physical Activity: Level 1 of the Physical Activity Pyramid

Lesson Vocabulary
CDC, FITT, NASPE, PCPFS, pedometer

▶ **www.fitnessforlife.org/middleschool/**
Click Student Info ▶ Topic 3.1

One type of activity in the Physical Activity Pyramid introduced in chapter 1 is lifestyle physical activity. Can you describe what lifestyle activity is? What lifestyle activities do you perform? How do lifestyle activities benefit you? When you finish this lesson, you'll know the answers to these questions. You'll also know about the FITT formula and some guidelines for participating safely in physical activity.

What Is Lifestyle Physical Activity?

In chapter 1 you were introduced to lifestyle physical activities. This type of physical activity is placed at level 1 of the Physical Activity Pyramid because it has many benefits and because it's easy for people of all ages to perform. Among adults, it's the most common form of physical activity.

The name "lifestyle activity" was chosen by experts to recognize the health benefits of activities of daily living. Lifestyle activities can be done by anyone. However, level 1 of the pyramid includes activities other than walking to school and working in the yard. In fact, level 1 includes all activities that are moderate—meaning equal in intensity to brisk walking—rather than those that are light or vigorous. For example, it includes moderate sports such as bowling and golf, and moderate recreational activities such as fishing. So although this book uses the term "lifestyle activity" to mean activities at level 1 of the pyramid, remember that all moderate activities are part of level 1.

What Is the FITT Formula?

The letters in **FITT** help you remember the four parts of a formula for determining how much physical activity is enough.

- **F** stands for frequency, which is how often you should be active, or the number of days you should take part in physical activity each week.
- **I** stands for intensity, which is how hard you should exercise. Should it be light, moderate, or vigorous?

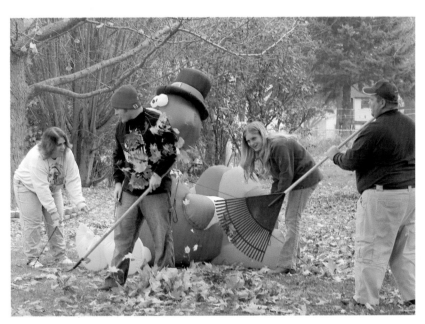

Moderate lifestyle activities are good for beginners and for people with limited activity choices.

- The first **T** stands for time, which is how long you should do your daily activities, or how many minutes you should be active each day.
- The final **T** stands for type. The many types of physical activity are described in the Physical Activity Pyramid in chapter 1 (see page 4).

Each type of physical activity from the first three levels of the Physical Activity Pyramid for teens has its own frequency, intensity, and time. For this reason, each type of activity has its own FIT formula. The final T is not needed because the activity's type is already known. The type of activity to be discussed in this chapter is lifestyle activity.

How Much Lifestyle Physical Activity Do I Need?

Several reports have described the physical activity needs of youth. A report of the National Association for Sport and Physical Activity (**NASPE**) indicates that youth need at least 60 minutes and up to several hours of physical activity each day. The Centers for Disease Control and Prevention (**CDC**) also recommend 60 minutes of activity for youth. The CDC is a U.S. government agency charged with protecting the health of citizens. Finally, a group of several hundred experts developed physical activity guidelines for teens. This group recommends that teens get both moderate and vigorous activity on a regular basis. This kind of activity should typically make up half of your total physical activity each day. On days when you do no other form of physical activity, you should do at least 60 minutes of lifestyle activity. But whether you do 30 minutes, 60 minutes, or more, you can spend the minutes continuously or spread them out over several activity periods lasting 10 minutes or more.

Table 3.1

FITT Formula for Lifestyle Physical Activity

F = Frequency	Perform lifestyle physical activity on all, or most, days of the week. Teens should be active a minimum of five days per week.
I = Intensity	Moderate; equal in intensity to brisk walking. Your heart rate goes up a bit but not as much as it does in vigorous activity.
T = Time	At least 30 minutes per day.
T = Type	Lifestyle and other moderate physical activities

FIT FACT

The American Heart Association and the American Cancer Society recommend at least 60 minutes of daily physical activity for teens to enhance lifelong health.

Based on the recommendations of experts, we can describe the amount of lifestyle physical activity teens need by using the FIT formula (see table 3.1).

If you're involved in active sports and recreation, you might meet the recommendation for physical activity (at least 60 minutes a day) without even counting your lifestyle physical activity. However, as you move into adulthood, you might not participate in active sports and recreation as frequently as you do now. Adults are more likely to participate in moderate lifestyle activities than other activities in the Physical Activity Pyramid. If you have not yet found an active sport or recreational activity to do on a regular basis, you might need to use lifestyle physical activity to secure some of the activity minutes you need each day to reach the recommended level.

Click Student Info ▶ Topic 3.2

Rest or inactivity

Exercise for flexibility

Exercise for strength and muscular endurance

Level 1 Active aerobics

Active sports and recreation

Lifestyle physical activity
F = All or most days of the week
I = Moderate (equal to brisk walking)
T = 30 or more minutes

Lifestyle or moderate physical activities are the base of the Physical Activity Pyramid.

Why Is Lifestyle Physical Activity at the Bottom of the Pyramid?

As noted at the beginning of this chapter, one reason lifestyle activity is at the bottom of the pyramid is that it's a very basic type of activity that most people can do. Many people with limitations that keep them from doing more vigorous activities can walk or do some other moderate physical activity that is equal to brisk walking. For example, people who rely on a wheelchair to get from place to place can navigate in their chair (wheelchair walking), as it qualifies as a lifestyle activity. Walking can be done by most people of all ages, including very old people. Other activities equal in intensity to brisk walking (such as taking the stairs rather than an elevator, doing yard work or other work around the house, or having an active occupation) count as moderate lifestyle activities. You can do these activities throughout your life.

A second reason lifestyle physical activity is at the bottom of the pyramid is that it provides many benefits for all people. Of course, it's best to do all types of activity from the pyramid each week. However, if for some reason you're limited in the types of activity you can perform, moderate activity is a good choice. For example, if you get injured, if you get sick, or if you're away from home and have little opportunity to be active, you can do moderate lifestyle activity. It can be done anywhere and with little equipment. It's a good starting point for beginners and for those who are getting back to exercise after an injury or illness. Because it's a basic type of activity, it fits well at the base of the pyramid.

The Pedometer

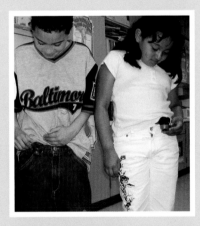

A **pedometer** is a computerized device that counts every step you take. You place it on your belt and wear it throughout the day to measure the amount of moderate activity you're getting. Each morning you push a button that sets the pedometer to zero, and each evening you read the number of steps on the pedometer and record it in an activity log. If your school has pedometers, you might be able to test one out to see how many steps you take each day. Because pedometers count all the steps you take each day, if you do both lifestyle activity and vigorous activity, you won't know how much of each type you performed. You may want to record more details about your activities or reset your pedometer before and after activities of different types.

Different groups recommend different numbers of steps per day for students. Since being active every day is important, the President's Council on Physical Fitness and Sports (**PCPFS**) offers a President's Active Lifestyle Award for people of all ages. It is meant to encourage people to be active every day by providing a way to record their activity and by offering awards for those who are active over a six-week period. You can count the time you're active, or you can count the number of steps you take each day using a pedometer. While this program was created in the United States, the step counts and amounts of time necessary to earn awards are appropriate for people in other countries as well.

Click Student Info ▶ Topic 3.3

Moving Together:
Safe Physical Activity

You might know about safety precautions, but do you follow them? Which precautions do you follow? Do you wear seatbelts every time you're in a car? Do you also wear appropriate safety gear when in-line skating or riding your bike? Do you follow traffic safety rules when walking and biking? Do you remember to warm up before and cool down after playing sports?

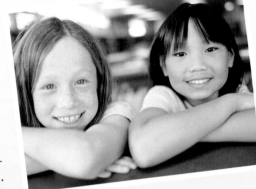

LaVerne and Katie decided that they wanted to be more active. They decided to meet three days a week after school to be active together. They planned to do several different activities on different days: running, in-line skating, swimming, biking, and tennis. Occasionally, they planned to join some other friends to play volleyball. Before beginning, they wanted to be sure that their activities would be safe.

Discussion Questions

1. Before beginning their first day's activity, how can LaVerne and Katie get ready for their activities?

2. What safety factors should LaVerne and Katie consider before they perform the activities they are planning?

3. What factors in the environment should LaVerne and Katie consider?

4. When playing sports or games with others, what can the girls do to ensure the safety of others as well as themselves?

Guidelines for Safe Participation

Being physically active is important to good health, but safety precautions are important. Consider the following factors when preparing for participation in physical activity.

▸ *Be medically ready.* Before beginning a new program, especially if it is very active, you should be certain that you are medically ready. Experts have developed a questionnaire called the PAR-Q that is sometimes used to determine medical readiness. Your teacher can help you determine your medical readiness using the PAR-Q.

▸ *Warm up before and cool down after your workout.* The warm-up gets your body ready for activity. It can help prevent injury and may improve your performance. The cool-down can help you recover after activity. For more on warm-ups and cool-downs, see page 6 in chapter 1.

▸ *Consider the weather.* If you're active outdoors, wear sunscreen. On hot days, dress properly and drink lots of water. Take frequent breaks and stop if you get too hot or feel dizzy or sick. In cold, wet, or windy weather, wear protective clothing. If the conditions are bad (such as too hot and humid, or too cold and windy), postpone activity or perform it indoors.

▸ *Wear protective gear when necessary.* Activities such as biking require a helmet; in-line skating requires a helmet and hand, elbow, and kneepads. Other activities also require special equipment. Find out what the appropriate protective equipment is for each activity you are going to try and learn to use it properly.

▸ *Get instruction and practice the activity to avoid accidents or falls.* When you learned to ride a bike, you likely got help and practiced to prevent falls. Good instruction and practice can help you avoid injuries in activities such as in-line skating and rock climbing.

▸ *Adhere to safety rules.* Some activities have rules to ensure your safety. For example, swimming in certain areas is prohibited because it can be dangerous. Diving in a shallow pool is against the rules for your protection.

▸ *Consider the safety of others.* A fast runner may want to jog more slowly when joining a friend who is a beginner. A beginner who tries to keep up with a more advanced runner may get blisters, become sore, and not have fun. In sports and games, take steps to ensure the safety of others by playing under control and having respect for other competitors.

▸ *Choose a safe play area.* Not all playgrounds are safe. Identify safe play environments in your area.

Click Student Info ▸ Topic 3.4

How Much Lifestyle Activity Do Most Teens Get?

Now that you know about how much lifestyle physical activity teens need, it might be interesting to see how much activity teens actually get. A national survey is done each year to see how many teens do at least five days a week of moderate lifestyle physical activity. Studies show that less than 30 percent of teens get enough lifestyle physical activity each week. Among boys, 27 percent get enough moderate physical activity each week, and only 23 percent of teen girls get enough. Preteens get more moderate activity than teens do, and young teens (13 to 14) get more moderate activity than older teens do (15 to 18). Do you get enough lifestyle activity each week? Are you more active than the typical teen?

Click Student Info ▶ Topic 3.5

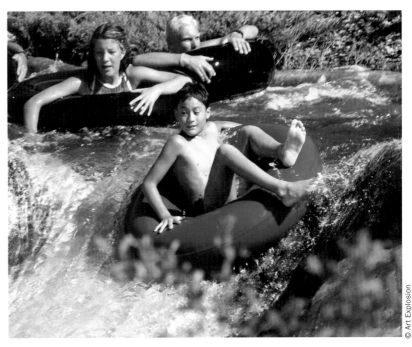

Fun recreational activities of moderate intensity are considered lifestyle activities.

Take It Home

Making Changes

Nobody's perfect. Some people eat too much junk food. Some have other bad habits. Some people aren't as active as they should be. Many people want to change what they do, but changing behavior can be difficult. To make a change, you need to know where you are before you start and where you want to go. If you're planning to take a trip, you look on the map for your starting place and then get directions to the place you want to go. You do something similar when you want to change a behavior. You need to know where you are when you start. Then you can decide how to get where you want to go.

So where do you stand when it comes to physical activity? How about friends and family? Where do they stand? When it comes to physical activity, people range from couch potatoes to active exercisers.

- Couch potatoes are inactive with no plans to become active.
- Inactive thinkers are inactive but thinking about becoming active.
- Planners are taking steps to become active.
- Activators are active but not on a regular basis.
- Active exercisers are active on a regular basis.

People are at different stages for all types of health behaviors, including eating, health habits such as brushing teeth and flossing, and bad habits such as smoking. Some are not thinking of change and some already have good health habits. If you're already active, maybe you can help a friend or family member become more active. If you're not an active exerciser, maybe friends and family can give you the support you need in order to become more active.

Use the worksheet supplied by your teacher to keep track of the different kinds of activities you perform on a typical day. Then use the information to see if you're getting the right amount of activity.

Lesson Review

- ▶ What is lifestyle activity, and what are some types of lifestyle activity?
- ▶ What is the FITT formula?
- ▶ How much lifestyle physical activity should teens perform?
- ▶ Why is lifestyle activity at the first level of the pyramid?
- ▶ What are some guidelines for participating safely in physical activity?
- ▶ How much lifestyle activity does the typical teen get?

Benefits of Lifestyle Physical Activities

Lesson Vocabulary
friction

Click Student Info ▶ Topic 3.6

When you do lifestyle activity, you get health and wellness benefits. Can you describe some of these benefits? What about physical fitness? Does lifestyle physical activity improve your fitness? When you finish this lesson, you'll know the answers to these questions. You'll also understand the importance of friction to your performance in physical activity.

Does Lifestyle Activity Improve My Health and Wellness?

Experts recommend lifestyle and other moderate physical activity for several different reasons. First, regular moderate lifestyle activity contributes to good health by improving the way some of the important body systems function. It helps keep the fat levels in the blood low, it helps blood pressure to stay at healthy levels, and it helps in maintaining a healthy body weight.

Lifestyle physical activity also helps people to resist common diseases such as heart disease, diabetes, and cancer. These are mong the leading causes of death in our society. Although teens are less likely to develop these diseases than adults, diabetes has become more prevalent in teens in recent years, and changes in body systems that lead to deadly diseases begin early in life. Lifestyle activity can help resist these changes.

Improved wellness is another benefit of moderate lifestyle physical activity. Having good wellness means that you can function effectively in daily living and that you feel and look your best. Performing lifestyle physical activities can also provide evidence of personal accomplishment. For example, doing yard work at home helps the family, and doing yard work as a part-time job can provide income for teens. Moderate lifestyle activities don't build high levels of physical fitness the way that activities from levels 2 and 3 of the pyramid do. However, for those who are low in fitness, especially cardiovascular fitness, lifestyle physical activities can help move a person into the healthy fitness zone.

A final but very important reason for doing lifestyle physical activity is that it's easy to perform as part of normal daily life by people of all ages and abilities. You can walk to school, work in the yard, ride your bike, and climb stairs without having special skills. Anyone can do it! People who do lifestyle activity get many benefits compared to those who are inactive. You get extra benefits if you do more activity than the recommended amount, such as vigorous physical activity or additional lifestyle physical activity. However, the biggest increase in benefits comes from doing the recommended amount of lifestyle activity, which dramatically increases health and wellness benefits. These benefits come with relatively little effort because lifestyle activities are easy to do.

Click Student Info ▶ Topic 3.7

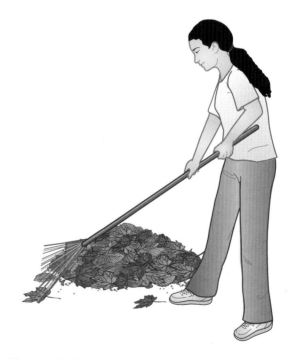

Lifestyle physical activities have many health benefits.

Biomechanical Principles: Friction

To produce movement, some friction often is necessary. For some activities, it is helpful to increase friction while for others it is helpful to decrease friction.

Friction is a force caused by one surface rubbing against another. The force of friction resists slipping between the two surfaces. Friction is important in physical activity for two reasons: slipping and gripping. In activities such as walking and running, gripping is necessary to get you going, to help you change directions, and to keep you from slipping. For lifting and holding objects and for activities such as rock climbing, gripping is good and slipping is not so good. In activities such as skiing and ice-skating, slipping is good and gripping is not so good. Likewise, slipping is good when you are pushing or dragging objects across the floor.

There are different ways to increase friction when it's needed or to reduce friction when it's not needed. Here are four examples:

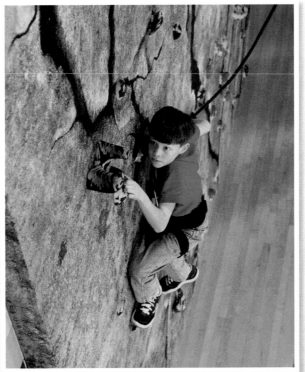

Using chalk to prevent slipping helps to increase your grip while climbing.

▶ Friction is increased when the surfaces that rub together are rough or irregular rather than smooth. Rubbing two pieces of rough sandpaper creates more friction than rubbing two pieces of regular paper.

▶ The harder you press two objects together, the more friction you create. Weight creates pressure, so sliding a heavy object along a floor is harder than sliding a light object.

▶ Applying a slippery substance to the surface of an object can decrease friction. For example, wet or greasy surfaces have less friction than dry surfaces.

▶ Applying substances that prevent slipping can increase friction. For example, gymnasts use a chalky substance on their feet to keep them from slipping on the balance beam.

You can use the information about friction to aid you in performing various activities. Rock climbers want friction in order to resist slipping movements of their hands along the rocks. They can increase friction and improve their grip by grabbing a rough rock rather than a smooth one, or by grabbing a dry rock rather than a wet one. They can get more friction and a better grip if they press their fingers against the rock more tightly. This means that improving your grip strength is important for better rock-climbing performance. Climbers also use special powders on their hands to increase friction.

In normal daily activities, you also can benefit from knowing about friction. When trying to turn a doorknob or hold a bottle upright, you don't want your fingers to slip. You can tighten your grip to increase the friction force. In walking or running, you need friction between your shoes and the ground so that your feet can push against the ground to move you forward or to help you turn without slipping. Running tracks often have a rough surface and shoes have a tread to increase friction and grip for running and turning. The deck of a boat should have rough surfaces to reduce your chance of slipping when the deck gets wet.

In some activities, you don't want a lot of friction. Skiers want to reduce friction between the snow and their skis so they can slide down the hill easily. The snow is smooth and wet. The skis may be waxed to reduce friction and increase sliding. Skiers also lift their feet slightly to reduce the friction between the snow and the skis when trying to turn the skis. Then they push down harder to get enough friction to be able to change directions. Of course, if there is too little friction because the ski slope is packed with ice, it may be too slippery to ski safely. Even in skiing, some friction is good, particularly for changing directions and slowing down.

Click Student Info ▶ Topic 3.8

When you push or pull a heavy object across the floor, it will move more easily if you reduce friction. You can reduce friction by putting the object on something smooth, like a carpet square, and making sure the floor is as smooth as possible. You can also reduce the force pressing the object downward by reducing its weight. For example, when moving a desk, you can remove the drawers or the contents of the drawers. You can also reduce friction by pulling up on the object to reduce its weight on the floor.

Friction is a force that affects the movement of many different kinds of objects. For this reason it relates to Newton's laws of motion. You may want to review these laws by visiting the *Fitness for Life: Middle School* Web site (see page 11).

Applying the Principle

To use friction in order to move effectively, you need to know when friction is good and when it's not so good. You also need to understand the factors that can increase or decrease friction. If you're walking on ice or driving on a wet road, you may not have enough friction to be able to start, slow down, or turn. Instead, you might slip, which could be very dangerous. In these activities, you would like to increase friction if possible, perhaps by spreading sand on the surface to make it rougher or by using shoes or tires with rough surfaces. You could also use weight to increase friction. Some people place a heavy weight in the trunk of their cars in the winter to increase the weight over the rear wheels of the car so the tires will be less likely to slip in the snow.

Some dancers need to slide gracefully across the floor, so they wear shoes with smooth soles to reduce friction. If you're trying to slide down a snowy slope, open a sliding door, or raise a window, friction can make it hard to accomplish your goal. In these cases, you would like to reduce friction. Do you know any tricks people use to decrease friction to accomplish these tasks?

Principle in Practice

Walk around in a circle, changing speeds. Think about the way your feet might slip as you do this. What are you doing when you feel your foot is most likely to slip? In order for you to push against the ground in any direction (to start, turn, or stop), your foot must have enough friction not to slip.

Practice holding an object, such as a book, between your thumb and fingers. First try holding the object when it's wrapped in slick paper. Then try holding the object when it's wrapped in a rough cloth. Notice how you need friction to prevent gravity from making the object slip through your fingers. What do you do to increase or decrease friction when holding each object? Which object is easier to hold between your fingers—the one with rough sides or the one with smooth sides?

Look at the soles of different shoes to see if they're likely to have much friction with the floor. Try dragging them across the floor to see if you can feel the difference in friction (resistance) you predicted. What kind of activities would each pair of shoes be good for?

Use the worksheet supplied by your teacher to look at how you can increase and decrease friction in two physical activities.

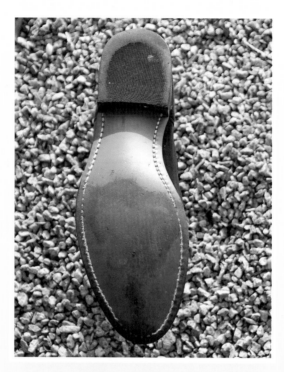

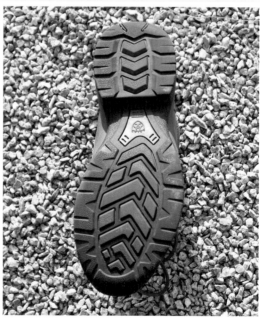

A shoe with a smooth sole (top photo) reduces friction on a surface such as snow, while one with a rough tread (bottom photo) can increase friction.

Does Lifestyle Activity Improve My Fitness?

Lifestyle activity is good for increasing health and wellness, but it's not one of the best types of activity for building physical fitness. Moderate activities can help low-fit people to improve and get into the healthy fitness zone in some areas, but they're not as good as more vigorous activities for building high-level fitness. As you'll learn in later chapters, you'll need to do activities from level 2 of the Physical Activity Pyramid to build cardiovascular fitness, and activities from level 3 of the pyramid to build strength, muscular endurance, and flexibility. Activities from the first three levels of the Physical Activity Pyramid will help you to maintain a healthy body fat level and a healthy body weight. Moderate lifestyle activities are especially good for controlling body fatness because you can do them for long periods of time without getting tired.

FIT FACT

Students who walk to school accumulate more steps per day than those who ride in a car or bus. Students who participate in after-school physical activities accumulate more steps per day than students who don't participate.

As you learned in chapter 1, teens are generally more active than adults. This is especially true for more vigorous activities at level 2 of the pyramid. However, it's not true for moderate activity. Adults do more moderate activity than teens. If teens do a lot of activity from levels 2 and 3 of the pyramid, it's OK for them to do less moderate activity. As mentioned earlier, however, doing regular moderate lifestyle activities early in life can help to develop habits that last a lifetime.

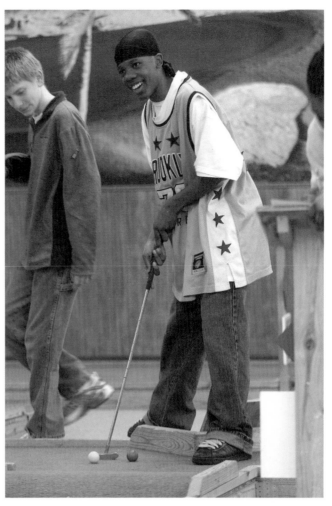

Moderate lifestyle activities enhance wellness by helping you feel good and enjoy life.

Lesson Review

▶ How does lifestyle physical activity improve your health and wellness?

▶ How is friction important to performance in physical activity?

▶ How does lifestyle physical activity improve your physical fitness?

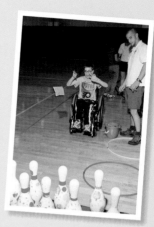

Chapter Review

Number your paper from 1 to 5. Read each question. After the number for the question, write a word or a phrase that best answers the question. The page number where you can find the answer is listed after the question.

1. In the FITT formula, what does the letter F stand for? (page 27)
2. Which government group works to prevent and control diseases in the United States? (page 28)
3. According to this chapter, what is the minimum number of minutes of physical activity that teenagers need daily? (page 28)
4. What is the name of a type of small computer that you can attach to your waist to count the number of steps you take? (page 29)
5. What is the name of the questionnaire used to help people decide if they're medically ready for physical activity? (page 30)

Number your paper from 6 to 10. Next to each number, write the letter of the best answer.

6. intensity
7. type
8. moderate activity
9. raking leaves
10. friction

a. refers to different kinds of activity
b. force caused by two surfaces rubbing together
c. a kind of lifestyle physical activity
d. activity equal in intensity to brisk walking
e. an indicator of how hard an activity is

Number your paper from 11 to 15. Follow the directions to answer each question or statement.

11. What is the FITT formula, and why is it important?
12. Explain why lifestyle physical activity is placed at the bottom of the Physical Activity Pyramid.
13. Give examples of guidelines for being safe in physical activity.
14. Give examples of how friction can help or hurt performance in physical activity.
15. Give examples of some of the benefits of lifestyle physical activity.

Ask the Author

Why does this book sometimes use FITT and other times use FIT?

Get the answer and ask your own questions at the *Fitness for Life: Middle School* Web site.

Click Student Info ▶ Topic 3.9

Unit Review on the Web

You can find unit I review materials on the *Fitness for Life: Middle School* Web site.

Click Student Info ▶ Topic 3.10

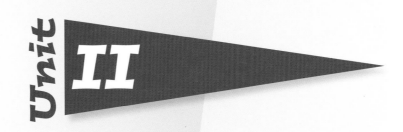

Aerobics, Sports, Recreation, and Flexibility Exercises

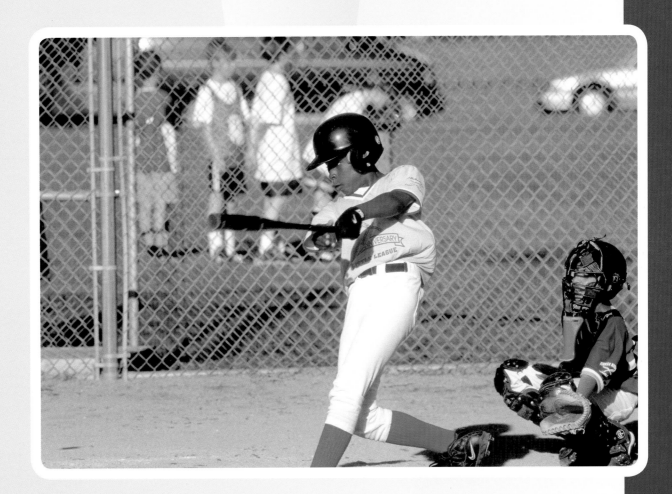

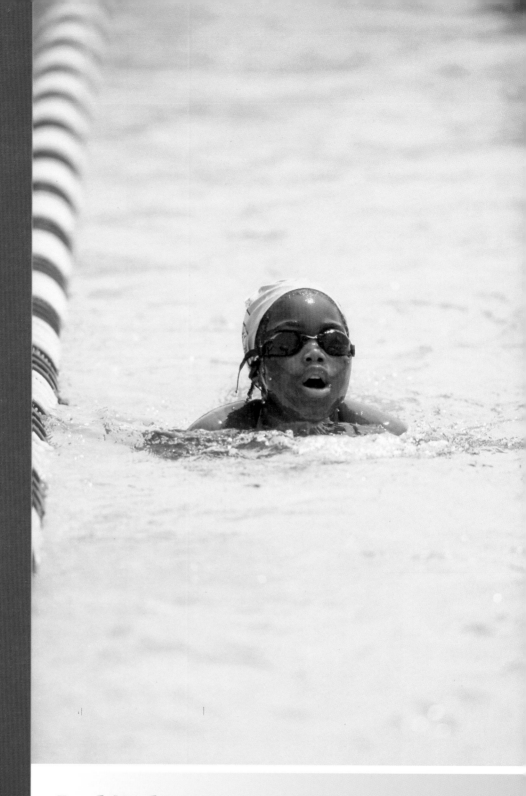

4

Active Aerobics

Active Aerobics: Level 2 of the Physical Activity Pyramid

Lesson Vocabulary

active aerobics, anaerobic, body image, resting heart rate, self-esteem, target zone

▶www.fitnessforlife.org/middleschool/
Click Student Info ▶ Topic 4.1

One of the types of activities in the Physical Activity Pyramid is called **active aerobics.** Do you know what *aerobics* means? What are some types of active aerobics? How much active aerobics do you need? Do you perform active aerobic activities? When you finish this lesson, you'll know the answers to these questions. You'll also know some guidelines for building self-esteem in physical activity and other situations.

What Is Active Aerobics?

Whether you're active or resting, your body needs oxygen to do its work. The air that you breathe contains oxygen. The oxygen that enters through your nose and mouth is carried to the lungs, where it's picked up by the blood. The blood is pumped by the heart through the blood vessels to all parts of the body including your muscles. The energy for activity is created when oxygen combines with simple sugars.

Click Student Info ▶ Topic 4.2

Your heart is a very important muscle. It uses some of your body's energy to pump oxygen-rich blood to all parts of your body. When you're inactive, your heart beats about 60 to 80 times per minute. This is called your **resting heart rate.** If you don't already know how to determine your resting heart rate, visit the *Fitness for Life: Middle School* Web site to get the necessary information.

Click Student Info ▶ Topic 4.3

Resting heart rates vary from person to person. As noted above, typical resting heart rates for teens vary from 60 to 80 beats per minute, but for some people, resting rates lower than 60 or higher than 80 are healthy. Resting heart rate, by itself, isn't a good indicator of physical fitness, but your resting heart rate is typically lower when you're fit than when you're unfit. Some very fit athletes have heart rates as low as 35 to 50 beats per minute. However, some very fit people don't have especially low heart rates compared to other people, and some unfit people have relatively low heart rates compared to others. This is because heredity affects heart rate as does age, body size, and health status.

When you begin physical activity, your heart beats faster than it does when you're inactive. This is because your body needs more oxygen. When you're active, your heart pumps more often to supply your body with the blood and oxygen that it needs. The harder you exercise, the more your heart rate increases.

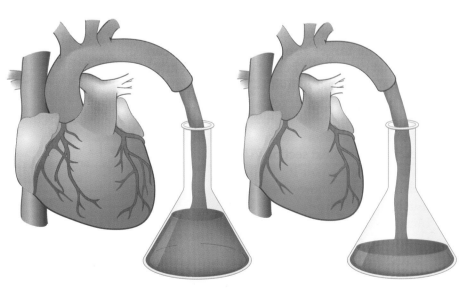

With regular exercise, the heart gets stronger and pumps more blood (left) than a less fit heart (right).

Moving Together: Building Self-Esteem

What does *self-esteem* mean? Do you think you have high or low self-esteem? Can you remember a situation that lowered your self-esteem? How did you feel in that situation? When you think about yourself, what do you feel good about? What do you think would improve your self-esteem?

Self-esteem is a term used to describe your feelings about yourself. Your self-esteem is affected by all of the things you do. For example, being a good student, artist, musician, or athlete; being fit; or doing well in social situations all contribute to good self-esteem. Different people are good at different things, so different people depend on different things to feel good about themselves. Your physical self-esteem is affected by your skills, your fitness, and your feelings about your body. Having high self-esteem means that you feel good about yourself for the things you can do well and that you don't feel bad if you don't do everything well.

Adrianna isn't especially lean and athletic, and she is self-conscious about her body. But she is a very talented artist. She avoids activity because she worries that she won't do well.

Jeremiah is good at basketball and also at schoolwork. His friends are on the basketball team, but they're not so good at schoolwork. Jeremiah sometimes doesn't want others to know that he gets good grades because he's afraid that his friends might not accept him socially. Sometimes he feels bad when others kid him about being a "brain."

Olivia does OK in school, but she isn't on any teams or in any special groups such as the band. She has a lot of friends because she is fun to be around and is supportive of her friends.

Charlie didn't do well on his physical fitness test. He was so disappointed that he told others that he wouldn't even try the next time he took the test. But he told himself he wished that he could do better.

Discussion Questions

1. Which of the teens do you think have high self-esteem?
2. What suggestions do you have for the teens you think have low self-esteem?
3. Do you have to be good at everything to have high self-esteem?
4. Does what the teens think about themselves matter in determining self-esteem?

Guidelines for Improving Your Self-Esteem

▶ *Focus on personal strengths.* Nobody is good at everything. But everybody is good at something. Focusing on your positive points builds self-esteem.

▶ *Think positively.* Some experts say that it's what you think that counts. That means that people who think positively about themselves have high self-esteem, even if they're not as good as other people in certain areas. Thinking negatively is not productive and can hurt your self-esteem. If you aren't good at something you would like to be good at, the best thing you can do is practice. If you need help, don't be afraid to ask for it.

▶ *Avoid unfair comparisons with others.* Too many people make unfair comparisons. For example, they might compare their performance in sports to that of a pro athlete or compare the way they look to the way movie stars look. Most movie stars don't actually look the same in real life as they do on the screen, and many pro athletes have problems just as other people do. Being the best you can be is better advice than trying to be like someone else. Even on fitness tests, try to meet the healthy fitness level rather than worry about how you compare with others.

▶ *Focus on things that are possible to change, and use your time wisely.* There are some things that you can't change and others that you must work hard to change. You can't change your height, your age, or even your basic physical features. But hard work can help you change some things. You can improve your skills, your fitness, and your body composition with regular physical activity. You can improve in your schoolwork if you study. You can improve your skills in art and music with effort and practice. Creating a schedule that gives you time for practice, time for regular exercise, and time to study will ensure that you'll improve in these areas. Avoid wasting time on things that you can't change or that won't lead to positive change.

▶ *Build your skills and fitness.* **Body image** is a part of self-esteem that refers to how you feel about your body. Eating well and doing regular physical activity can provide the fitness to enhance your body image and self-esteem. Good nutrition and regular exercise can also help you build muscle and maintain a healthy body weight. Building skills through practice can help you feel good about yourself physically. People who accept their bodies and try to build on what they have are more likely to have a good body image than those who worry about what they don't have or can't do.

▶ *Respect the confidentiality of personal information.* Personal information is just that—personal. Because good health and self-esteem are important goals, fitness test results and other personal information should go only to the person being tested or others with whom he or she wants to share them. Making results public can lead to unfair comparisons such as those described earlier. When doing fitness self-assessments such as those you will do later in this book, it's best to work with a friend who agrees to keep your results private.

▶ *Find friends who provide support, and be supportive of friends.* Having friends can boost self-esteem. To have friends, you must be a good friend. Support those whom you care about. Help those who need your support. True friends don't act friendly only when they want others to do things for them.

▶ *Ignore unfair comments.* Unfortunately, not all people are supportive. Sometimes people can make unfair and negative remarks that hurt the feelings of others. People sometimes make negative comments when they're frustrated or when they're trying to boost their own self-esteem by hurting others. But this technique doesn't really boost self-esteem. In fact, people who make unfair comments often have low self-esteem, and their unfair comments may even make it lower. It's hard to ignore negative comments because we all prefer compliments. However, sometimes we read negative things into other people's remarks unfairly because of our own insecurities. It's best to expect that other people have good intentions. This stops you from reading negative feelings into innocent or well-meant remarks.

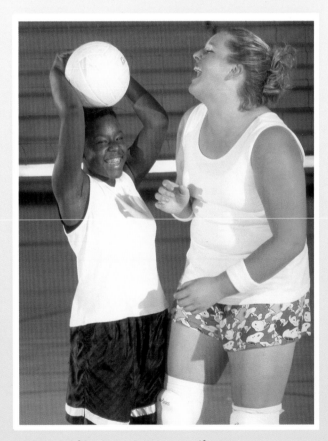

Having good friends can boost your self-esteem.

Click Student Info ▶ **Topic 4.5**

Table 4.3

Active Aerobic Activities

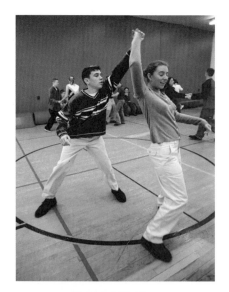

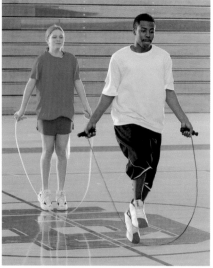

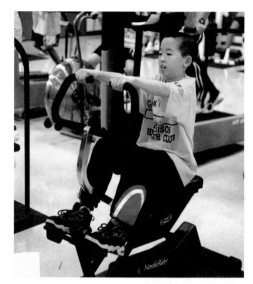

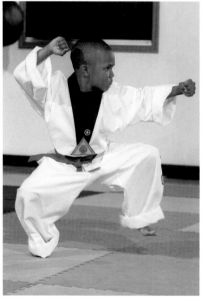

Active aerobics includes many different kinds of activities. The key is getting your heart rate into the target heart rate zone. Some lifestyle activities (such as biking) are active aerobics when done vigorously. Some active sports (such as swimming) and active recreation activities (such as in-line skating and skiing) can also be considered active aerobics if performed so the heart rate is in the target zone.

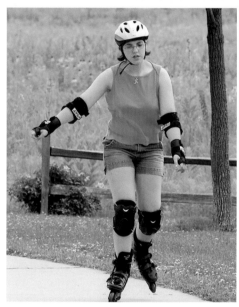

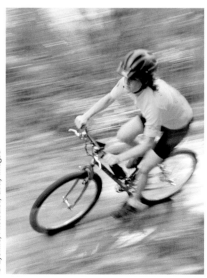

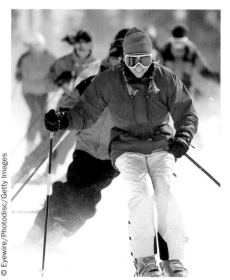

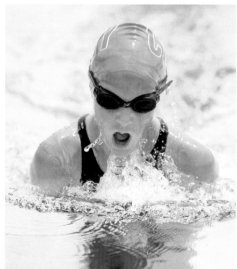

© Eyewire/Photodisc/Getty Images

© Eyewire/Photodisc/Getty Images

Anaerobics

If your body can supply enough oxygen to keep you going, you're doing aerobic activity. If you elevate your heart rate into the target zone, you're doing active aerobic activity. But if your activity is so vigorous that your heart rate is elevated above the target zone, you're doing anaerobic activity.

Anaerobic activities are so vigorous that your body can't supply enough oxygen to keep you going for long periods of time. When you perform an activity at maximum intensity, such as when you swim as fast as you can, you can continue the activity for only 30 to 40 seconds before you have to stop and rest. Anaerobic fitness is needed to perform well in many sports that require bursts of anaerobic activity, but it's not necessary for good health. If you plan to play a sport and want to learn more about anaerobic exercise, you can consult with your teacher or a school coach.

Click Student Info ▶ Topic 4.6

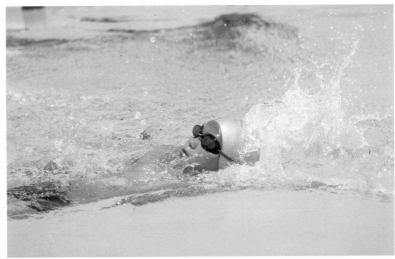

Swimming as fast as you can is an example of anaerobic activity.

FIT FACT

Aerobic means "with oxygen." In aerobic activity, the body is supplied with enough oxygen to keep going for a long time. *Anaerobic* means "without oxygen." In this book, *anaerobics* refers to activities (such as sprinting) for which the body can't supply enough oxygen to keep going for a long time.

Take It Home

Tuning In

"How are you?" You probably hear that question a lot. You hear it from people you haven't seen in a long time and even from people you just talked to yesterday. Often people answer the question with "I'm fine." You can't tell every person all of the details of how you're doing when they ask, but you can learn to understand more about how you're doing by "tuning in to" or "listening to" your body. If you listen, your body can tell you many things. For example, you can tell whether or not you've been active by counting your heartbeats, monitoring your breathing, and noticing the feeling of sweat. If you've been very active, your muscles will tell you the next day because they may be sore. This is especially true if you do an activity that you don't normally do.

Your body can tell you when you're cold by shivering and when you're hot by sweating and increasing body temperature. Pain can also be your body's way of telling you that you're injured or ill. Your body gives you signals when you're tired and when you need sleep. Your stomach grumbles when you're

hungry. Sometimes you feel emotions that cause your body to react.

In many of the activities you do in this unit, you'll need to pay attention to both your body and your feelings. What is your heart doing? What makes this activity easier or harder? When do you feel good? What makes you feel bad? Use the worksheet supplied by your teacher to tune in to your body before, during, and after physical activity.

Lesson Review

- ▶ What are active aerobics, and what are some types of active aerobic activities?
- ▶ How much active aerobics do you need?
- ▶ Describe the best type of active aerobics for you, and give reasons for your choice.
- ▶ Describe some guidelines for building self-esteem in physical activity.
- ▶ What is anaerobic activity, and what are some examples of anaerobic activities?

Benefits of Active Aerobics

Lesson Vocabulary
center of gravity, PACER, stability

Click Student Info ▶ Topic 4.7

When you do active aerobics, you get health and wellness benefits. Can you describe some of these benefits? Do you know what cardiovascular fitness is? How can you tell whether you have good cardiovascular fitness? When you finish this lesson, you'll know the answers to these questions. You'll also understand the importance of stability to your performance in physical activity.

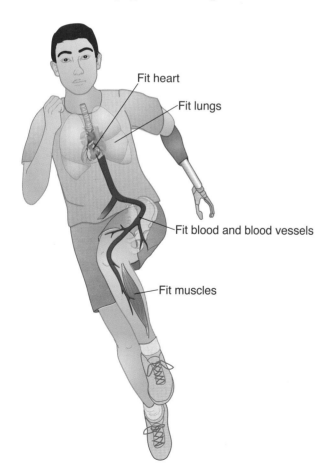

Fit heart

Fit lungs

Fit blood and blood vessels

Fit muscles

Cardiovascular fitness requires fitness of many body systems.

Why Should I Do Active Aerobics?

Active aerobic activities produce many of the same health and wellness benefits of lifestyle physical activities. One major benefit that you get from active aerobics that you can't get from moderate lifestyle physical activity is cardiovascular fitness. In fact, active aerobics is probably the best method of building good cardiovascular fitness. As you learned in chapter 1, cardiovascular fitness is the ability of your heart, lungs, blood vessels, and blood to work efficiently and to supply the body with oxygen. Cardiovascular fitness allows you to do physical activity for a long time without getting tired. Some of the benefits of having good cardiovascular fitness are described in the following paragraphs.

Cardiovascular Fitness and Sports

Teens interested in playing a sport should be very interested in active aerobics because most sports require good cardiovascular fitness and active aerobics is a good way to get it. Sports such as cross country running, track and field, skiing, swimming, soccer, and tennis are just a few that require cardiovascular fitness. You can't perform your best in sports unless you do activities that build good cardiovascular fitness.

Click Student Info ▶ Topic 4.8

Cardiovascular Fitness for Health

Teens who do lifestyle physical activity get health benefits such as a reduced risk of developing certain diseases. Teens who also do active aerobics get similar benefits and more! Active aerobics can help you get out of the low fitness zone and into the healthy fitness zone for cardiovascular fitness.

Cardiovascular Fitness and Wellness

Active aerobics and the cardiovascular fitness that it produces help you to feel and look your best by burning calories and keeping off body fat. You'll feel your best because you'll be less tired. Best of all, you'll have fun because you'll be participating in activities that you enjoy.

Cardiovascular Fitness and Safety

In some special cases, people have needed to run to get help, shovel sand into sandbags, or even shovel snow for long periods of time. Good cardiovascular fitness would help a person to perform activities such as these.

Cardiovascular Fitness for Work

Certain jobs require cardiovascular fitness. For example, to get a job as a member of a fire or police department, you need good cardiovascular fitness. Park rangers, lifeguards, construction workers, ranchers, farmers, fitness instructors, and members of the military all must have good cardiovascular fitness. Any job that requires you to work for long periods of time and that causes your heart to beat fast requires good cardiovascular fitness.

Click Student Info ▶ Topic 4.9

FIT FACT

When you begin exercising, the blood vessels to your exercising muscles expand, and the blood vessels to your stomach and intestines contract. This increases the blood flow to your working muscles.

How Do I Know if I Have Cardiovascular Fitness?

There are many different ways to assess your cardiovascular fitness, including tests such as the mile run, the step test, and the walking test. Visit the *Fitness for Life: Middle School* Web site for more information on some of these tests.

Click Student Info ▶ Topic 4.10

In this section you'll learn how to assess your cardiovascular fitness using the **PACER** test. The PACER is part of the Fitnessgram National Physical Fitness Test and is a fun way for teens to assess their cardiovascular fitness.

Once you have taken the PACER test, you can determine your fitness rating using table 4.4 for males or table 4.5 for females (see p. 50).

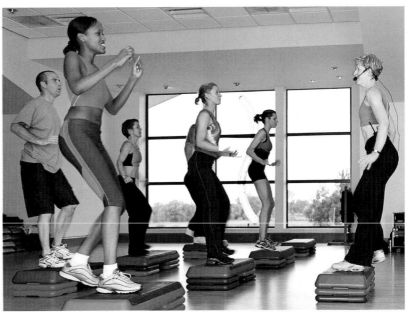

© Bananastock

Aerobic dance instructors and lifeguards must have good cardiovascular fitness.

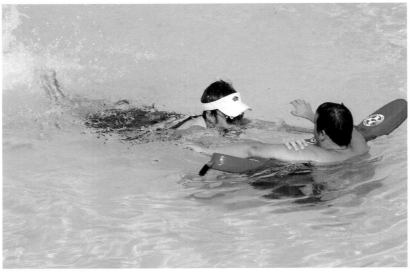

Biomechanical Principles: Stability and Balance

Stability and balance are important for success in many physical activities, but sometimes instability is necessary to allow you to move and perform various physical activities.

Stability is the ability of an object to maintain its balance. If an object loses its balance, it will fall. Humans must have stability to stay in balance even when standing still. In physical activity, you need to have stability and you need to stay in balance. For example, you need good stability and balance when playing defense in basketball, when receiving a serve in tennis, and when performing activities such as in-line skating and skiing.

Many factors can affect your stability and cause you to lose your balance. If someone pushes against you, such as in wrestling, practicing judo, or playing football, it can cause you to lose your balance. Turning or changing direction quickly can make you lose your balance. Slipping because of too little friction can cause balance problems. A strong wind can also cause instability.

There are some things you can do to improve your stability. First, you can spread your feet to have a wider base of support. When babies learn to walk, they do it with their feet wide apart. If you learned to ski or skate, you probably did the same thing.

The second thing you can do to improve your stability is to lower your **center of gravity.** Your center of gravity is the center of your body weight. If you bend your knees, you lower your center of gravity and will have improved stability.

The third thing you can do to improve stability is to keep your center of gravity (the center of your weight) over the center of your base of support. When a basketball player is playing defense and wants to stay in balance, the feet are spread apart, the knees are bent to lower the center of gravity, and the head and shoulders are centered between the two feet.

The three stacks of cans shown below may help you to understand stability and balance while standing still. The white dots in the stacks of cans show the center of gravity.

▶ Stack A has a wide base. It's also lower to the ground and has a lower center of gravity. The center of gravity is over the center of its base, so this stack is quite stable.

▶ Stack B has a narrow base and has a higher center of gravity. It's less stable than stack A.

▶ Stack C is much less stable than the other two stacks. Stack C has a narrow base and a high center of gravity, and the center of gravity is not over the base, so this stack of cans would fall unless you held it in place.

○ center of gravity

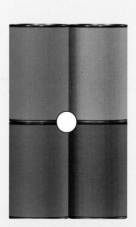

Stack A is quite stable.

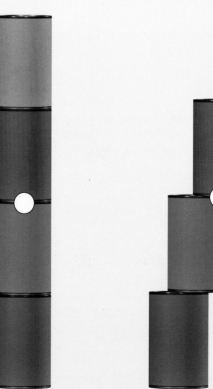

Stack B is less stable.

Stack C is the least stable.

Biomechanical Principles: Stability and Balance *(continued)*

To be stable in physical activity, you should be more like stack A than stack B or C. This is particularly important when you don't want to lose your balance because of a force that pushes against you.

Although stability is important when performing many kinds of activities, there are times when you want to be unstable. When you want to start moving, you need to lean in the direction of movement. This means that your center of gravity will be in front of your base of support if you want to move forward. For example, a sprinter in the starting blocks is preparing to move forward. Having her center of gravity forward will help her to get out of the starting blocks quickly when it's time to start because her feet are back against the starting blocks, and her center of gravity is in front of her feet. In fact, the sprinter actually falls out of the starting blocks to get a quick start. When the starting gun fires, she just lifts her hands off the ground and is instantly leaning forward. This position allows the greatest possible push back against the starting blocks for the fastest possible start. The same kind of instability is also necessary when changing directions, which you often do in sports.

Applying the Principle

Which of the following activities require stability and which require instability? Describe how a person can increase or decrease stability in each activity. Also discuss how your need for stability or instability may change in each activity.

- Playing defense during a basketball game
- Starting a sprint
- Walking on a balance beam
- Skiing downhill
- Carrying a food tray with one hand above your shoulder

Principles in Practice

How can you change the width of the base of your body and the location of your center of gravity to be more stable and to be in balance? Practice movements for several different activities to be stable and more balanced.

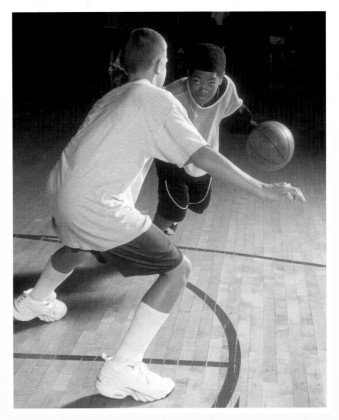

Good stability is important when playing defense in basketball.

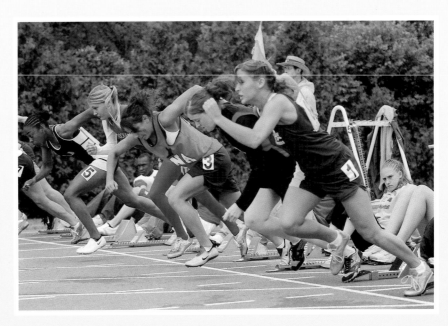

The body is unstable (leaning forward) when starting a race.

Click Student Info ▶ Topic 4.11

Your goal for cardiovascular fitness and the PACER test is to get in the healthy fitness zone. If you fall below the healthy fitness zone, you should consider increasing your cardiovascular fitness. Those in the healthy fitness zone may want to do regular active aerobics to move to a higher level in the zone. Scores above the healthy fitness zone may be beneficial to those interested in athletic and other types of performance, so if you want to be an elite athlete, go for it. However, it's important to understand that scores above the healthy fitness zone aren't necessary to achieve the many benefits described earlier in this chapter.

PACER Test

PACER stands for Progressive Aerobic Cardiovascular Endurance Run and is a test of cardiovascular fitness. You'll need a tape or CD player and a special tape or CD to perform the test. Because the test requires this special equipment, it might not be as easy to do as other cardiovascular assessments. However, by taking this test you can see whether you meet the national health-related cardiovascular fitness standard. The objective of the test is to run back and forth across a 20-meter distance as many times as you can.

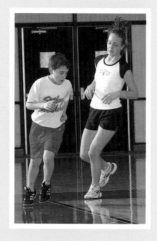

1. When you hear the beep on the tape, run across the 20-meter area and touch the line before the tape beeps again. Turn around.

2. At the sound of the next beep, run back to the other side. (You must wait for the beep before running.) The beeps will come faster and faster, causing you to run faster and faster. The test is finished when you twice fail to reach the opposite side before the beep.

3. Your score is the number of times you can run the 20-meter distance before your test is finished. Record this number on your worksheet. Then find your fitness rating in table 4.4 or table 4.5.

Table 4.4

PACER Ratings for Males

Age	Needs improvement	Healthy fitness zone
10	22 or fewer	23–61
11	22 or fewer	23–72
12	31 or fewer	32–72
13	40 or fewer	41–72
14	40 or fewer	41–83
15+	50 or fewer	51–94

Measured in laps.
Reprinted, by permission, from C. Corbin and R. Lindsey, 2005, *Fitness for life, 5th ed.* (Champaign, IL: Human Kinetics), 123.

Table 4.5

PACER Ratings for Females

Age	Needs improvement	Healthy fitness zone
10	14 or fewer	15–41
11	14 or fewer	15–41
12	22 or fewer	23–41
13	22 or fewer	23–51
14	22 or fewer	23–51
15+	22 or fewer	23–51

Measured in laps.
Reprinted, by permission, from C. Corbin and R. Lindsey, 2005, *Fitness for life, 5th ed.* (Champaign, IL: Human Kinetics), 123.

Lesson Review

▶ What are some of the benefits you get from performing active aerobics?

▶ What is cardiovascular fitness, and how can you tell if you have it?

▶ What are some of the benefits of having good cardiovascular fitness?

▶ How is stability important to performance in physical activity?

4

Chapter Review

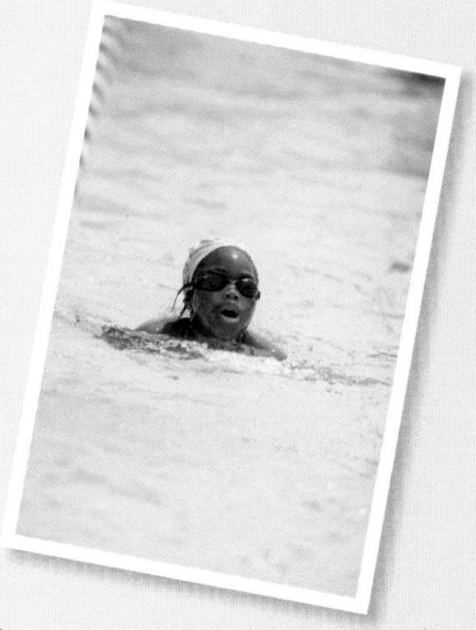

Number your paper from 1 to 5. Read each question. After the number for the question, write a word or a phrase that best answers the question. The page number where you can find the answer is listed after the question.

1. What term describes the number of times your heart beats when you're sitting and doing nothing? (page 39)

2. At what level of the Physical Activity Pyramid do you find active aerobics? (page 40)

3. How many days a week should you do active aerobics? (page 40 or 41)

4. How long should each active aerobics exercise period last? (page 41)

5. Which type of health-related fitness is best built by doing regular active aerobics? (page 46)

Number your paper from 6 to 10. Next to each number, write the letter of the best answer.

6. jogging
7. energy
8. target zone
9. stability
10. PACER

   a. results from combining oxygen and simple sugars
   b. a test of cardiovascular fitness
   c. ability to maintain balance
   d. heart rate just right for aerobic activities
   e. a type of aerobic activity

Number your paper from 11 to 15. Follow the directions to answer each question or statement.

11. Explain the difference between aerobics and active aerobics.

12. Give examples of good active aerobic activities.

13. Give examples of guidelines for building self-esteem.

14. Describe some of the benefits of active aerobics.

15. Give examples of the need for stability in performing physical activity.

Ask the Author

How can I help my parents have better cardiovascular fitness?

Get the answer and ask your own questions at the *Fitness for LIfe: Middle School* Web site.

Click Student Info ▶ Topic 4.12

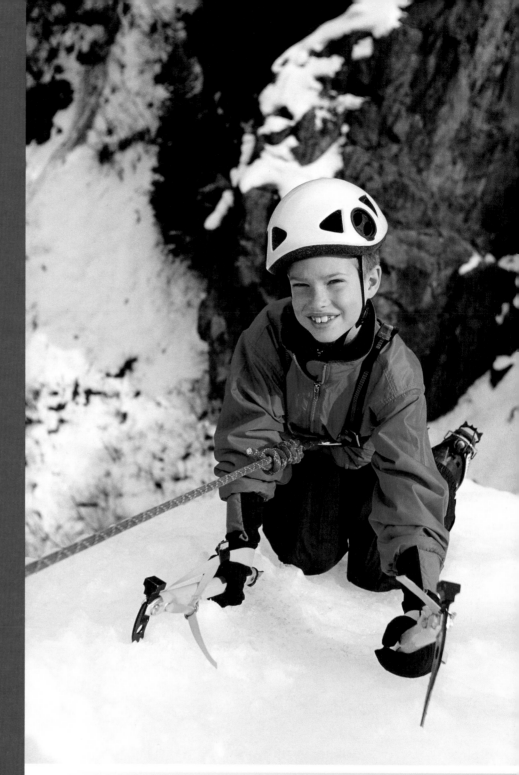

5

Active Sports and Recreation

Lesson 5.1

Active Sports and Recreation: Level 2 of the Physical Activity Pyramid

Lesson Vocabulary

active recreation, active sports, anaerobic, games, lifetime sports, participation sports, physical recreation, recreation, spectator sports, sports, strategy, tactics

▶ **www.fitnessforlife.org/middleschool/**

Click Student Info ▶ Topic 5.1

Two types of activities in the Physical Activity Pyramid are active sports and active recreation. Do you know what active sports are? Do you know what active recreation is? What are some types of active sports and recreation? Do you perform active sports and recreation? When you finish this lesson, you'll know the answers to these questions. You'll also know some guidelines for making sports and recreation more fun by following the rules.

What Are Active Sports?

You have probably played many different sports, but it may be hard for you to describe exactly what makes a physical activity a sport. **Sports** are physical activities that use the large muscles of the body. Sports have well-defined rules and typically involve competition between individuals or teams. Sports have winners and losers. Sports also typically require a **strategy** (an overall plan) and **tactics** (specific plans to meet your goals).

Chess and card games are typically not considered sports because they don't use the large muscles of the body. **Games** that don't have well-defined rules and that aren't highly competitive, such as children's games, aren't considered sports even though they use large muscles.

Sometimes a sport can be done as a form of active recreation. For example, one person

might run cross-country as a competitive sport, while another person might run long distances not for competition but as a form of active recreation.

There are several kinds of sports. Some are quite vigorous and get the heart to beat faster than normal, and others are less vigorous and are more similar to lifestyle activities. Vigorous sports are often called **active sports.** Soccer and tennis are examples of active sports.

Golf and bowling are examples of less vigorous sports. They're similar in intensity to moderate lifestyle activities such as walking, gardening, and housework. These less active sports, like lifestyle activities, have health benefits but aren't especially good for building cardiovascular fitness. As you'll learn later in this chapter, active sports are a good way to build cardiovascular fitness.

Some sports are more popular than others. Sports that many people perform on a regular basis are considered **participation sports.** Some sports are called **spectator sports** because many people watch them on TV or in person. Sometimes a sport can be both a participation sport and a spectator sport. For example, you might play baseball and also enjoy watching it.

Sports in which many people participate at all ages are considered **lifetime sports.** All sports have benefits, but it's better to learn active lifetime sports that you can participate in both now and as you grow older. Choosing an active sport is a good idea because you get both health and cardiovascular benefits if you do the sport regularly. Table 5.1 classifies some of the most popular sports in our society. The table also rates the popularity of sports by different age groups.

Click Student Info ▶ Topic 5.2

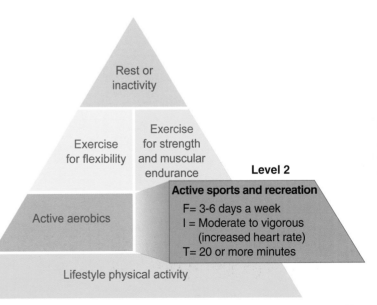

Active sports and active recreation are at level 2 of the Physical Activity Pyramid.

As indicated in table 5.1, sports are often classified as individual sports or team sports.

- Individual sports are those that you can do by yourself or as an individual. For example, you can play golf by yourself. Tennis is also considered to be an individual sport even though you need at least one other player to play a game. One advantage of individual sports is that they're easier to do for a lifetime because you need at most only one other person to play.

- Team sports require other players. Softball, basketball, and soccer are examples of team sports. Team sports are very popular with people of school age because schools and communities offer many opportunities. One disadvantage of team sports among adults is that there might be fewer community teams for adults, so it might be difficult to get enough people together to have a game.

Sometimes people who play individual sports are also members of teams. For example, several golfers can form a team. In tennis if you play doubles, you team up with another person. Even if you play alone against one opponent, scores from individual matches can earn points for the tennis team.

Active sports often require you to do vigorous physical activity for short bursts followed by periods of rest. For example, in basketball you might run up and down the court quickly three or four times and then stop for a free throw or a time-out. If you jog up and down the court, you're doing aerobic activity. If you run fast, you're doing **anaerobic** activity, which means that you're using

Table 5.1

Characteristics of Popular Sports

Sport	Active	Team	Individual	Popular with kids	Popular with teens	Popular with adults	Lifetime
Archery			✓				✓
Badminton	✓		✓				✓
Baseball		✓		✓ (P, S)	✓ (P, S)	✓ (S)	
Basketball	✓	✓		✓ (P, S)	✓ (P, S)	✓ (P, S)	✓
Bowling			✓			✓ (P, S)	✓
Extreme sports	✓		✓	✓ (P, S)	✓ (P, S)		
Field hockey	✓	✓					
Football	✓	✓		✓ (P, S)	✓ (P, S)	✓ (S)	
Golf			✓			✓ (P, S)	✓
Gymnastics	✓		✓	✓ (P)		✓ (S)	
Handball	✓		✓				✓
Hockey	✓	✓		✓ (P, S)	✓ (P, S)	✓ (S)	
Ice skating	✓		✓	✓ (P, S)		✓ (S)	✓
Skiing	✓		✓	✓ (P, S)	✓ (P, S)		✓
Soccer	✓	✓		✓ (P)	✓ (P)		
Softball		✓		✓ (P)	✓ (P)	✓ (P)	✓
Swimming	✓		✓	✓ (P)	✓ (P)	✓ (P)	✓
Tennis	✓		✓	✓ (P)	✓ (P)	✓ (P, S)	✓
Volleyball	✓	✓			✓ (P)		

A designation of popular is based on the number of people who typically perform this sport on a regular basis (P = participation) or watch this sport on a regular basis (S = spectator).

The "topspin" serve in tennis has a high bounce because the spin causes a downward curve that makes the ball hit the ground at a steep angle.

oxygen faster than your body can supply it. This is one reason you need to stop and rest every now and then. Even though sports such as basketball aren't truly aerobic, they can have the same benefits as active aerobic activities if your heart rate is kept in the target zone most of the time. So active basketball is a good way to build both health and cardiovascular fitness benefits. Tennis is another example of an active sport that requires bursts of vigorous activity followed by rest periods. When played actively, it builds both health and cardiovascular fitness.

Click Student Info ▶ Topic 5.3

What Is Active Recreation?

Recreation refers to activities that you do during your free time. The word *recreation* means to re-create, or to be refreshed. Painting, enjoying music, reading, acting, and playing games such as cards or chess are forms of recreation that aren't particularly physical. Recreation that uses the large muscles of the body is sometimes referred to as **physical recreation**. This type of recreation is done during your free time just for enjoyment and relaxation.

Physical recreation activities that are vigorous enough to get your heart to beat faster are forms of **active recreation**. Active recreational activities build cardiovascular fitness. Examples include cross-country skiing, orienteering, and kayaking. Many types of active aerobics (such as aerobic dance or jogging) and active sports (such as tennis and racquetball) could be considered active recreation because they can be done during your free time, they use the large muscles of the body, they're vigorous, and they're done for fun. However, this book uses the term "active recreation" to mean fun and vigorous physical activities that typically aren't competitive and aren't considered active sports or active aerobics. Some of the most popular forms of recreational physical activities are listed in table 5.2.

Table 5.2

Recreational Physical Activities

Activity	Is It Active?*
Backpacking	Often
Biking	Sometimes
Boating	Not often
Camping	Not often
Canoeing	Sometimes
Fishing	Fresh water—not often Deep sea—sometimes
Games, including new games	Sometimes
Hacky sack	Not often
Hiking	Often
Kayaking	Often
Orienteering	Often
Rock climbing	Sometimes
In-line skating	Often
Rowing	Sometimes
Skateboarding	Sometimes
Skating	Sometimes
Sledding	Sometimes
Skiing	Often
Swimming	Sometimes

*The way you perform an activity helps determine whether it is considered active.

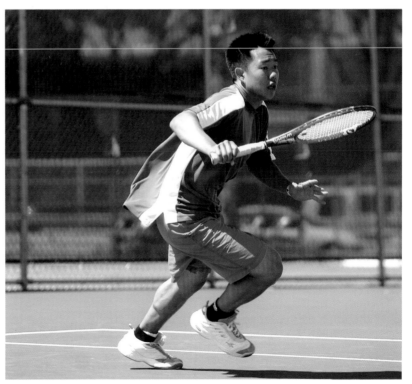

Active sports such as tennis require good cardiovascular fitness.

Moving Together: Following Rules

Have you ever played a game with someone who was cheating? How did it make you feel? What did you do about it? Would you break the rules in a game if no one would find out? Why or why not?

Several friends were discussing their experiences in sports. Julia told about playing in a school basketball game. Alexis, a player on the other team, was guarding her and kept hitting her in the arm every time she tried to shoot a basket. Julia felt that the referee didn't call every foul that Alexis committed. She considered fouling back to get even.

Phung described a situation in a baseball game when he was the catcher. A player on the other team slid into home just as the ball arrived. The umpire called the runner "safe," but Phung was sure that he had tagged the runner in time. He considered arguing with the umpire.

Max didn't play on a sports team, but he liked to go boating with his family. There were several rules for using the boat, and one rule was to wear your life jacket. Max felt that the life jackets did need to be in the boat, but he didn't want to wear one.

Discussion Questions

1. What advice would you have for Julia?
2. What advice would you have for Phung?
3. What advice would you have for Max?
4. Is it OK to violate the rules in some cases?
5. How can you control yourself and keep from being frustrated when others don't play by the rules?

Guidelines for Maintaining Self-Control

▶ *Play by the rules.* Sometimes it's hard to play by the rules when others don't, but if you play by the rules, your example may give others the courage to play fairly, too. It's true that some people won't follow the rules no matter what, but you can only control your own behavior, not the behavior of others.

▶ *Remember that umpires and referees make mistakes.* Sports officials are people just like everyone else. Even when they try hard, they make mistakes just like we make mistakes when we play sports. Over the long haul mistakes will balance out. Sometimes a bad call will go against you, but other times calls will be in your favor.

▶ *Retaliation often backfires.* Bad calls or unnecessary fouls sometimes lead to retaliation. Nearly everyone who has played sports has learned that retaliation rarely pays off. Not only is the person who retaliates likely to get caught and penalized, but when a person retaliates, he or she often feels bad and has less fun.

▶ *Arguing doesn't help you and leads to losing control.* Decisions have to be made in sports and games. If a referee or an umpire makes a decision, the players must agree to accept that decision. If there is no official, the players must learn to make group decisions themselves to avoid arguments. Arguing can cause you to lose your focus and perform poorly, and it might cause you to lose control of your temper.

Good Reasons for Following Rules

▶ *Rules are meant to make games fair.* Rules aren't always perfect, but if we all accept them and follow them, games will be more fun.

▶ *Rules keep people safe.* Many accidents result from ignoring safety rules and playing out of control.

▶ *Rules help officials and participants have self-control.* Because rules make games fair and safe, they help prevent people from getting angry and losing control.

Click Student Info ▶ Topic 5.4

Some forms of physical recreation, such as fishing and some forms of hiking, aren't especially vigorous. These activities can be considered moderate lifestyle physical activities similar to those described in chapter 3. Recreation doesn't always have to be active, but if cardiovascular fitness is your goal, the activity must cause your heart to beat in the target zone. Table 5.2 will help you to determine which recreational activities are active and which are not. You can tell the difference by paying attention to your heart rate and breathing while doing an activity.

As table 5.2 indicates, many recreational activities can be performed outdoors. For many people just being outdoors is relaxing because it gives them an opportunity to appreciate nature, such as leaves changing colors in the fall or snow drifting down in the winter. Recreational activities and sports vary from culture to culture. For example, people in colder parts of the world often choose winter activities such as skiing, sledding, and skating, and people in warmer parts of the world choose activities such as swimming and boating.

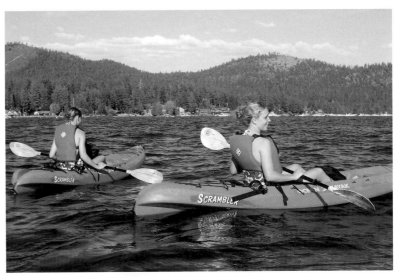

Take It Home

I Spy

"I would be active, but there's nowhere to go to do what I want to do." Have you ever heard a person say something like that? Have you ever said something like that? Can you find recreation, sports, and activity clubs in your community that interest you, your family, and your friends? Can you find parks or school playgrounds that are safe and have the equipment you need? Are there other places that you and others can go to be active? Are there safe places to walk that have good lighting and good sidewalks?

Knowing where to look and whom to ask about sports and recreation opportunities requires detective skills. Use the worksheet supplied by your teacher to investigate active sports clubs and active recreation clubs in your area. Your searches might lead to a lifetime of enjoyable activities.

Click Student Info ▶ Topic 5.5

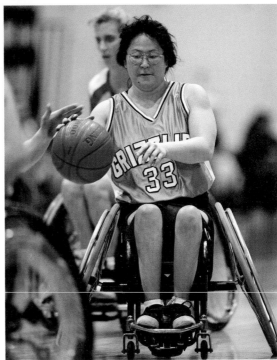

Active sports and recreation activities, such as kayaking or basketball, can be moderate or vigorous.

Lesson Review

▶ What are active sports, and how do they differ from games and other types of sports?

▶ What is active recreation, and how does it differ from other types of recreation?

▶ Name several sports. Are they team sports or individual sports? Are they spectator sports or participation sports? Are they most popular with kids, teens, or adults?

▶ Describe some guidelines for maintaining self-control and some good reasons for following rules when performing physical activities.

Lesson 5.2

Benefits of Active Sports and Recreation

Lesson Vocabulary

acceleration, deceleration, velocity

Click Student Info ▶ Topic 5.6

When you participate in active sports and recreation, you get health, wellness, and fitness benefits. Can you describe some of the most beneficial active sport and recreation activities? What are some of the best types of sports and recreation for you? When you finish this lesson, you'll know the answers to these questions. You'll also understand the importance of acceleration and velocity to your performance in physical activity.

What Are the Benefits of Active Sports and Recreation?

Sports have many benefits. Perhaps the best benefit is that they're fun. Even if you don't enjoy all sports, you probably have found several that you do enjoy. Even the least active sports and recreation activities provide health benefits similar to those provided by lifestyle physical activities. Active sports and active recreation have the added advantage of building cardiovascular fitness. This is one reason why active sports and recreation are included along with active aerobics in level 2 of the Physical Activity Pyramid. To gain cardiovascular fitness, you must follow the FIT formula that you learned in chapter 3. You must perform active sports and recreation for at least 20 minutes at least three days a week, and your heart rate must be elevated into the target heart rate zone.

FIT FACT

Sports and recreation activities can be adapted for people with disabilities. In "beep-beep softball," the ball makes a beeping noise so that people who are visually impaired can participate. In wheelchair tennis, a person in a wheelchair is allowed two bounces to get to the ball.

Sports and recreational activities can help you in many other ways as well. They can help you to relax and reduce the stresses in your life. They cause your body to expend calories that can help you maintain a desirable weight and feel and look your best. They provide a great way to meet friends and enjoy social interactions. They can help you learn to work as part of a team, which can benefit you in your adult career. Finally, participation in active sports and recreation can help you build parts of fitness other than cardiovascular fitness, including flexibility and muscle fitness. You'll learn more about these in later chapters.

Use the worksheet supplied by your teacher to interview other students about their favorite active sports and recreation activity. Ask them about the fitness benefits they gain, why they enjoy the activity, and what advice they can give to others who want to try the activity.

Click Student Info ▶ Topic 5.7

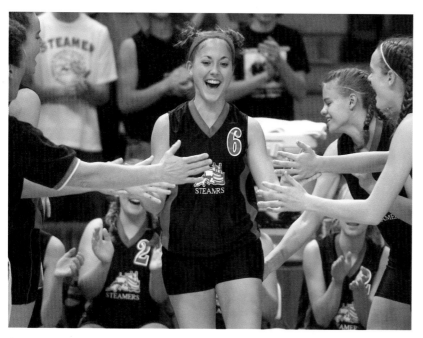
Active sports provide a way to meet friends and enjoy social interactions.

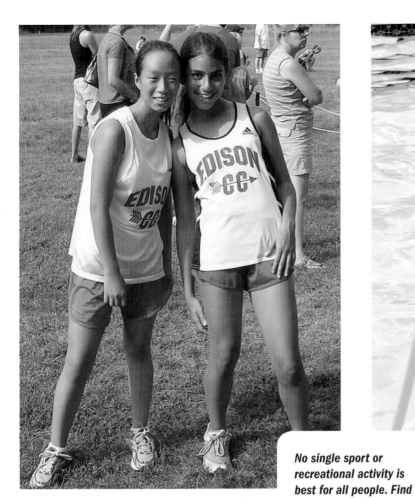

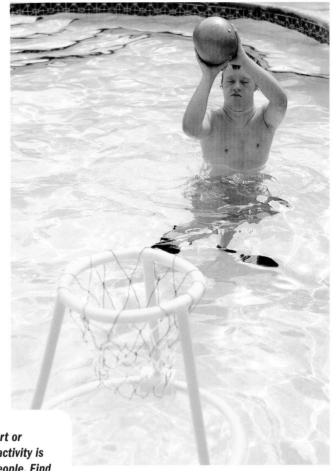

No single sport or recreational activity is best for all people. Find activities that you enjoy and that you'll do on a regular basis.

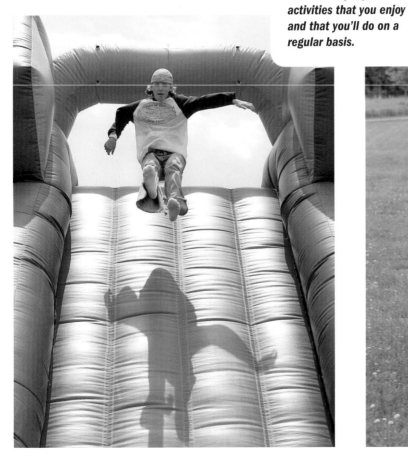

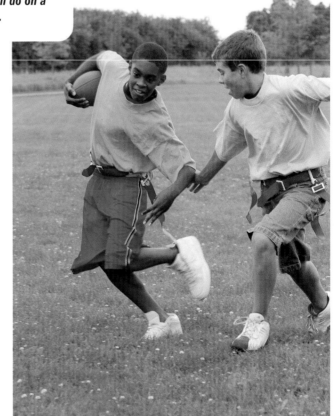

Biomechanical Principles:
Velocity, Acceleration, and Deceleration

Velocity, acceleration, and deceleration are important in the performance of physical activities, especially those that require speed and fast movements.

Velocity refers to the speed of movement. The term **acceleration** means causing an increase in speed (velocity) of a movement. **Deceleration** refers to a reduction in velocity. When a car moves away from a stoplight, it's accelerating. It continues to accelerate as long as its speed increases. The actual speed that the car is traveling at any point in time is its velocity. When it starts to slow down, it is decelerating.

Like a car, the body accelerates at the beginning of a race. The velocity of the body while running may be constant for a while, and then it decelerates after reaching the finish line. Runners with good acceleration and high velocity are fast runners.

The energy from food is used to contract the muscles to create force. The force causes the levers of the body to move. When the levers first begin moving, they cause acceleration. Acceleration requires a lot of energy. When a runner moves at a constant speed, energy expenditure is less than when accelerating.

Muscles can also be used to cause acceleration and high rates of velocity when using implements such as a baseball bat or a golf club. Good acceleration that results in fast bat speed or club speed allows you to hit a ball a long way. In fact, bat speed and club speed are more important than the heaviness of the bat or the club that you use. That is why metal bats and clubs are made with light metals. A light bat can be swung with high velocity, allowing a person to hit a ball a long distance.

Friction can affect the velocity of an object. For example, when a ball hits the ground, it slows down (decelerates) because of the friction created between the ball and the ground. Air resistance can also cause deceleration. For example, a strong headwind could slow the speed of a thrown ball.

Acceleration and velocity are important for good performances in some physical activities. Controlling movement during acceleration and high velocity is also important. For example, if you swing a bat too fast, you might lose control of the bat and fail to make good contact with the ball. When rollerskating or skiing, if you accelerate too fast and move at too high a speed, you might lose control and fall. You need good acceleration of your leg to kick a ball far, but it's also important to control your leg when it has high velocity to make sure that you contact the ball squarely.

For optimal performance, you should know when acceleration and high velocity are needed. You also need to know when to limit acceleration and velocity to control movements for optimal performance and safety. A reckless driver is one who accelerates too fast and drives too fast. In physical activity you sometimes need to accelerate as fast as possible and to travel at a high speed. Sometimes too much acceleration and velocity is reckless and may result in poor performances.

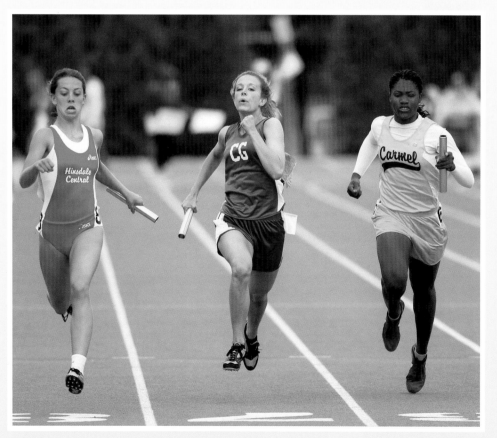

Runners accelerate at the beginning of a race, try to run at maximum velocity during the race, and decelerate after crossing the finish line.

Biomechanical Principles: Velocity, Acceleration, and Deceleration   *(continued)*

Applying the Principle

To move effectively, you need to know when to accelerate quickly and when to have high-velocity movements. This is true for total-body movements such as running, skating, and skiing. It's also true when using equipment such as a bat or a golf club, and for body levers such as those used when kicking and throwing a ball. Sometimes you want to throw a ball with maximum velocity—for example, throwing a fastball during a baseball game—but other times you may want to apply spin to cause the ball to curve. How might acceleration and velocity be needed in different ways for the following activities listed?

▶ Hitting a ball as far as possible

▶ Making sure you contact a ball in the center of a tennis racket

▶ Pitching a ball for accuracy

▶ Running as fast as possible

▶ Running so that you can change directions when needed

▶ Slowing down to avoid a collision in an activity

Principles in Practice

Velocity, acceleration, and deceleration are important for efficient and effective movement in normal daily activities. Controlling them is also important for safety when performing physical activities. Practice techniques that allow you to accelerate, decelerate, or maintain a constant velocity. Practice when moving your whole body (such as when running), when moving a piece of equipment (such as a tennis racket), and when using one of the levers of your body (such as throwing a ball with your arm).

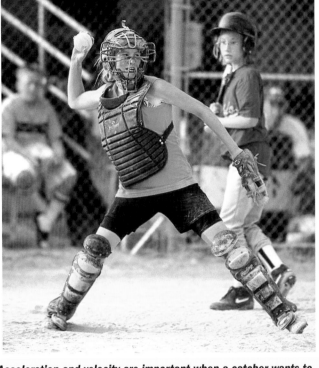

Acceleration and velocity are important when a catcher wants to throw out a runner who is trying to steal a base.

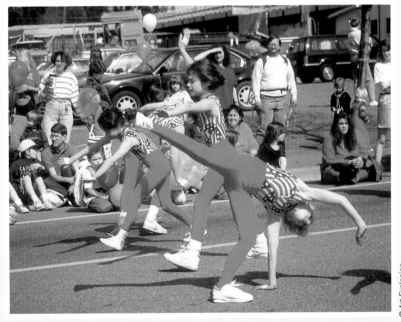

Performing gymnastics stunts requires acceleration and fast movements, but it also requires controlling body movements for safety.

© Art Explosion

Click Student Info ▶ Topic 5.8

What Types of Sports and Recreation Are Best?

There is no best sport or recreational activity for all people. What is fun for one person might not be as fun for another. Each sport and activity has its benefits. You should choose an activity that's fun for you and that provides benefits that are best for you.

Consider some of the following guidelines when choosing sport or recreational activities:

- *Select sports and recreational activities that provide benefits that you need.* For example, if you need to improve your cardiovascular fitness, choose an activity that causes your heart rate to increase.

- *Choose activities that match your abilities.* Teens with good cardiovascular fitness may choose soccer or cross-country running, and those with good flexibility may choose gymnastics or extreme sports (you can explore possibilities at the *Fitness for Life: Middle School* Web site).

- *Try many different activities.* By trying different activities, you can see which ones you like best and which ones match your abilities.

- *Choose activities that are accessible to you.* Be sure you have the space and equipment necessary to do the activity. If the activity is a team activity, you must have other people who are also interested in doing the activity.

- *Choose activities that you'll practice.* As you know, practice helps you develop good skills. Good skills help you perform better and make the activity more enjoyable.

- *Choose activities for which you can get good instruction.* Good instruction helps you understand how to use the biomechanical principles that you've learned, as well as other principles that affect the activity. This knowledge can help you practice better, learn better, and perform better.

FIT FACT

Based on estimates from the International Sports Federations, the most popular sports in the world are soccer, basketball, volleyball, and table tennis.

- *Consider activities that you can enjoy now and also later in life.* Being active should be a lifetime goal. Choose activities that you enjoy now, even if you may not do them later in life. But also choose activities that you enjoy now and that you'll be able to perform and enjoy in the years ahead.

Click Student Info ▶ Topic 5.9

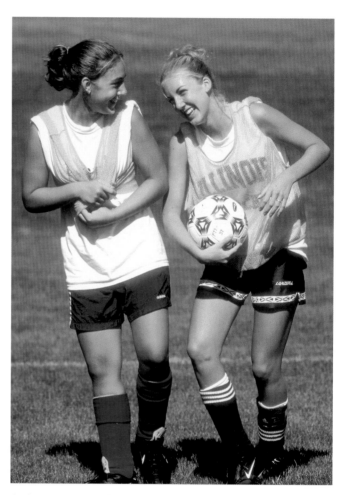

Active sports and active recreation are fun.

Lesson Review

- ▶ How do active sports and recreation improve your health, wellness, and fitness?

- ▶ How much do you need to participate in active sports and recreation to build cardiovascular benefits?

- ▶ How are acceleration and velocity important to performance in physical activity?

- ▶ What types of active sports and recreation are best for you?

5 Chapter Review

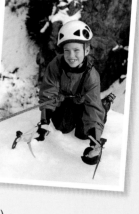

Number your paper from 1 to 5. Read each question. After the number for the question, write a word or a phrase that best answers the question. The page number where you can find the answer is listed after the question.

1. Which type of physical activity described in this chapter has rules, is competitive, and has winners and losers? (page 53)

2. What do you call sports that can be done by people of all ages? (page 53)

3. What do you call recreational activities that use the large muscles of the body? (page 55)

4. What word describes an increase in velocity (speed) of movement? (page 60)

5. What word describes a decrease in the velocity (speed) of movement? (page 60)

Number your paper from 6 to 10. Next to each number, write the letter of the best answer.

6. playing cards
7. kayaking
8. tennis
9. football
10. musical chairs

a. an example of a popular participation sport
b. an example of active recreation
c. an example of a popular spectator sport
d. an example of a game
e. an example of recreational activity that is not physical recreation

Number your paper from 11 to 15. Follow the directions to answer each question or statement.

11. How do recreation, active recreation, and physical recreation differ?

12. Give examples of why it's important to play by the rules and keep self-control when playing sports.

13. Give examples of some of the benefits of participating in active sports and recreation.

14. Give examples of guidelines for selecting sports and recreational activities that are best suited to your needs and interests.

15. Define velocity, acceleration, and deceleration, and give examples of how each is important in sports.

Ask the Author

If you want to play sports, is it better to specialize in one sport or to learn several different sports?

Get the answer and ask your own questions at the *Fitness for Life: Middle School* Web site.

Click Student Info ▶ Topic 5.10

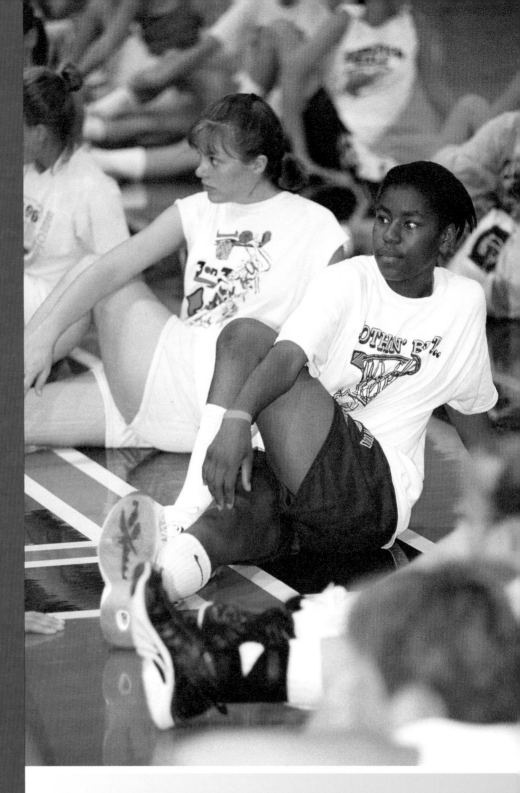

6

Flexibility Exercises

Lesson 6.1

Flexibility Exercises: Level 3 of the Physical Activity Pyramid

Lesson Vocabulary

ballistic stretching, gravity, joint, ligaments, muscles, PNF (proprioceptive neuromuscular facilitation), range of motion, static stretching, strain, strategy, tactics, tendons

▶ www.fitnessforlife.org/middleschool/
Click Student Info ▶ Topic 6.1

One of the types of activities in the Physical Activity Pyramid is flexibility exercise. Do you know what flexibility is? Do you know the best way to stretch your muscles to build flexibility? When you finish this lesson, you'll know the answers to these questions. You'll also know some guidelines that will help people to feel comfortable in physical activity and to make it more fun.

What Is Flexibility?

Flexibility is the ability of your joints to move as they're supposed to move. Each **joint** (location where your bones join together) in your body is designed to move in a certain way. The amount of movement in a joint is called its **range of motion.** Some joints, such as the hip and the shoulder, allow a large range of motion because they can move in many directions (see Biomechanical Principles on pages 73-74). Other joints, such as the knee and the elbow, bend in only one direction. So the amount of flexibility you have is affected by your joints.

Click Student Info ▶ Topic 6.2

Flexibility is also affected by other factors such as your age, your gender, and the structure of your bones. Most parts of health-related physical fitness improve with age. However, flexibility is the one part of physical fitness that decreases with age. Children are more flexible than most teens, and teens are typically more flexible than adults. Very old people are the least flexible of all. Girls and women typically have better flexibility than boys and men, though that's not always true. Other factors, such as the structure of your bones and the way the joints fit together, can affect flexibility. Some people have a joint structure that allows more range of motion than in other people who have joints with a tighter bone structure.

No matter how old you are, whether you're a male or a female, or what types of bones and joints you inherit, you can improve your flexibility by doing regular stretching exercises. All physical activities require some flexibility. For example, basketball requires long and fit **muscles,** especially in the legs. The girls in the photos below do regular stretching exercises, so they have good flexibility and good range of motion.

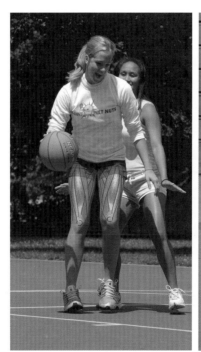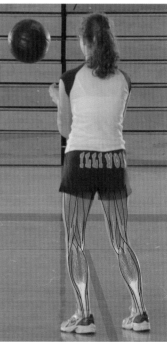

Regular stretching lengthens muscles that are used in physical activities.

How Do I Build Flexibility?

Some degree of stretching occurs naturally during lifestyle activities, sports, aerobic activities, and recreational activities. But often, it's not enough to build the flexibility you need for good health. Performing regular stretching exercises from level 3 of the Physical Activity Pyramid is the best way to build flexibility. It's important to know that you can have good flexibility in one part of your body without having it in another. For example, you could have long muscles and good flexibility in the lower part of your body but short muscles and poor flexibility in the upper part of your body. You should also know that incorrect stretching can be harmful and can result in joint or muscle injury (see Biomechanical Principles on page 73-74).

When you stretch your muscles, you also stretch your tendons. **Tendons** are the bands of tissue that connect muscles to bones. Both muscles and tendons are elastic, so stretching doesn't harm them if done properly. **Ligaments** attach bones to bones, but they're not elastic, so it's not good to overstretch them. Good stretching exercises, such as the ones described in this book, stretch muscles and tendons but don't stretch ligaments.

The most common type of stretching is **static stretching**. *Static* means "stationary" (without movement). When you perform static stretches, you stretch the muscle until it's longer than normal and then hold the stretch. Table 6.1 shows several ways to do static stretching.

Stretching is most effective when the muscles are warm. This is why a general warm-up (see page 6 in chapter 1) should be done before a stretching warm-up. Your regular stretching exercises that aren't part of a stretching warm-up should be done after a general warm-up or after you have done activities that get your body warm.

Another way to build flexibility is called **PNF (proprioceptive neuromuscular facilitation)**. When doing PNF, you contract your muscles before you statically stretch them. The contraction before the stretch helps the muscles relax so they can be stretched more easily. For example, before performing the second calf stretch exercise in table 6.1, contract your calf muscle by pushing your toes against the towel. Then pull on the towel to stretch the calf muscle. Visit the *Fitness for Life: Middle School* Web site for basic exercises for building flexibility using static stretching and PNF.

Click Student Info ▶ Topic 6.3

A third way to build good flexibility is **ballistic stretching**, a type of stretching used by athletes and very fit people. Instead of statically stretching the muscle, you bob or bounce to cause the muscles to stretch. Ballistic stretching isn't recommended for beginners. It's hard to control ballistic movements, which can result in applying too much force against a muscle and can lead to injury. You'll need the assistance of a coach or teacher to know when and how to do this type of stretching.

Click Student Info ▶ Topic 6.4

Level 3

Rest or inactivity

Exercise for flexibility

F = 3-7 days a week
I = Moderate stretch
T = 15 to 30 seconds, 1 to 3 times

Exercise for strength and muscular endurance

Active aerobics

Active sports and recreation

Lifestyle physical activity

Flexibility exercises are at level 3 of the Physical Activity Pyramid.

Table 6.1

Types of Static Stretches

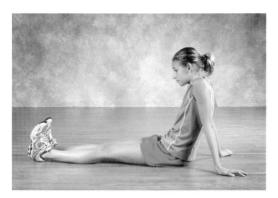

Self-assisted stretch with opposing muscles.

Contract the muscles of your shins to pull your toes forward and stretch your calf muscle.

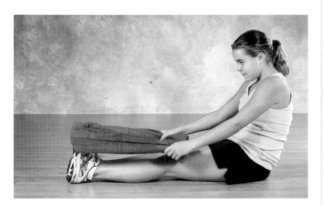

Self-assisted stretch with the use of arms and hands.

Loop a towel behind your toes and pull gently with your hands and arms to stretch your calf muscle.

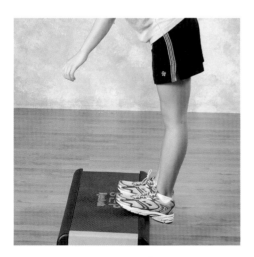

Gravity-assisted stretch.

Stand on a box or curb and let **gravity** force your heels lower than your toes, stretching your calf muscles.

Body-weight assisted stretch.

Lean forward, keeping your heel on the ground and stretching your calf muscle.

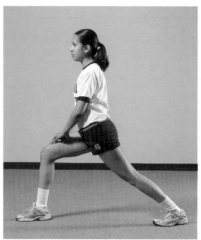

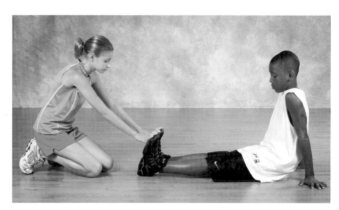

Partner-assisted stretch.

Have a partner push gently on your toes, causing your calf muscle to stretch. Partners need to communicate to avoid overstretching.

Note: Static stretches can be performed as PNF stretches by contracting a muscle or muscle group before you stretch it. For example, the girl doing the self-assisted stretch with the towel can push against the towel with her toes (contracting her calf muscles) before pulling with the towel to stretch her calf muscles.

Moving Together:
Feeling Comfortable in Physical Activity

There are many reasons why teens sometimes avoid participating in physical activity with others. They might be afraid of making a mistake and looking bad. They might want to avoid being teased by others who'd put down the activity by saying, "That's just for girls" or, "That's just for boys." They might have missed the beginning of the activity and think it's too late to join in. Do you sometimes feel uncomfortable in certain activities? Do your friends sometimes seem uncomfortable in activities that you enjoy? What can be done to make activities more comfortable for different people?

Tenzin, Sam, José, and Jasmine have learned a lot since they started the Fitness for Life program. They've learned about the many different parts of physical fitness and the different kinds of physical activity. They've begun to learn how to use practice to build the skills they need to do physical activities that they enjoy. But recently they became involved in a situation that made them uncomfortable.

On a weekend they planned to go to the park with friends from school. The four met at Tenzin's house so that they could walk to the park together. However, José said that he was going to go home because he didn't have what he called "fancy sports clothes" like some of the other teens who would be at the park. José's friends encouraged him to go with them.

The plan was to play a competitive game of volleyball. But before the game started, several problems occurred. Two boys started choosing teams, and many of the girls said they didn't want to play—they just wanted to watch. Some of the boys who were waiting to be picked said that they didn't want to play, either. Tenzin and Jasmine really wanted to play volleyball, but they decided to watch because so many other girls were watching.

Discussion Questions

1. What should Sam, Tenzin, and Jasmine say to José to encourage him to go with them? How might they help José feel OK when he arrives at the park?
2. What could the friends say to encourage all of the teens to participate in the game? How might Tenzin and Jasmine get involved? How might they help other girls get involved? How could the friends help José to get involved?
3. Are there actions other than talking that could be taken to help everyone get involved in the activity? What might these be?

Guidelines for Feeling Comfortable in Physical Activity

▶ *Talk about the activities you all enjoy.* Before you plan an activity, talk with all members of your group to learn which activities they enjoy.

▶ *Vary your activities.* If possible, choose an activity that everyone enjoys. That's not always possible, but you can agree to do different activities so that you'll eventually do an activity for everyone in the group.

▶ *Modify games.* Change the rules and equipment to make the game more fun for your group. For example, try using a larger, softer ball in place of an official volleyball. Or play two games with smaller teams rather than one big game. Forming new teams from time to time allows people to be team members with many different people.

▶ *Consider cooperative rather than competitive games.* Competitive activities can be fun if all people have similar skills. But if some members of the group don't have good skills, noncompetitive activities can be more fun. For example, play a game of volleyball in which the goal is to see how many hits in a row both teams can make together.

▶ *Avoid choosing sides in a way that causes some people to feel bad.* Having two people choose teams can cause hurt feelings, especially among those who get picked last. Check with your teacher about ways to choose sides so that teams are even without hurting anyone's feelings.

▶ *Practice some of the skills before playing the game.* If some group members have good skills, they can teach other group members and help them practice the skills. If all group members develop their skills, the activity will be more fun for everyone.

▶ *Choose an activity location where not many people are watching.* Some people are self-conscious when others watch them play. The activity might be more fun for everyone if you find a play area where other people aren't watching and commenting on your performance.

▶ *Do something after each activity to make group members want to try again.* Sitting down and talking in a social way can make people feel a part of the group. Even if someone isn't especially good at the current activity, he or she might stay in the group if being in the group is fun. Think of other things you can do to include all people in the group.

▶ *Encourage others, but don't overdo it.* Give words of encouragement to everyone in your group, but especially to those who don't have as much skill. But don't overdo it. If you give certain people too much encouragement, they might think that you feel sorry for them because of their skills.

▶ *Consider the way you dress.* If some members of the group are unable to dress in special clothing, especially if that clothing is expensive, you might want to dress down a bit. This can help others feel more comfortable in the group.

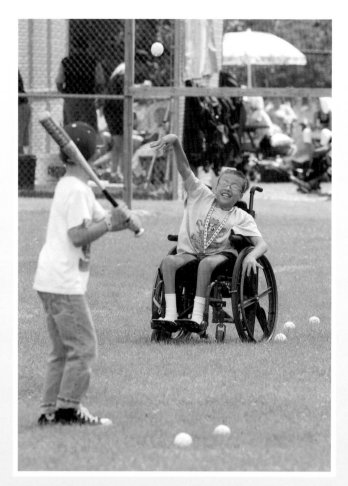

Give all players a chance to develop their skills.

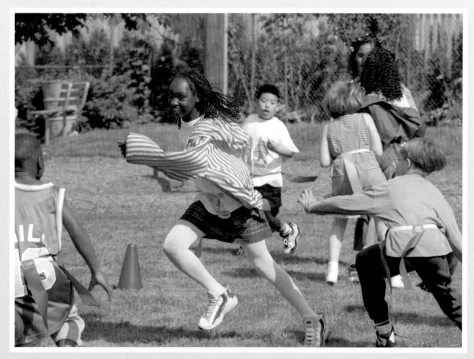

Modifying games can be a way to make them fun for everyone.

Click Student Info ▶ **Topic 6.5**

How Much Stretching Is Enough?

You already know that a muscle must be stretched beyond its normal length for it to get longer. But how far should you stretch a muscle? If you stretch it too little, it won't grow longer. If you stretch the muscle too far, you could injure it. For example, athletes sometimes stretch a muscle too much, causing a muscle injury called a **strain.** For best results you should follow the FIT formula for flexibility.

The FIT formula for static stretching and PNF is shown in table 6.2.

Before you stretch specific muscles, it's important to get the muscles warm. To get warm, you can do a general warm-up as described in chapter 1 (page 6) or start your workout with moderate activities before doing the stretching part of your workout. It's also important to cool down after your workout by doing moderate activities and stretching.

Table 6.2

The FIT Formula for Muscle Fitness for Teens

Flexibility exercises	Static stretching	PNF
Frequency	Stretch daily if possible; if not, at least three days a week.	Daily if possible; if not, at least three days a week.
Intensity	Stretch so that you feel tension in the muscle and even a slight burning sensation, but you should not feel pain.	Contract the muscle to be stretched (10 seconds), and then stretch as described for static stretching.
Time	Hold each stretch 15 to 30 seconds. Perform one to three times. Rest at least 10 seconds after each stretch.	Hold each stretch 15 to 30 seconds. Perform one to three times. Rest at least 10 seconds after each stretch.

Take It Home

TEAM (Together, Everyone Achieves More)

"We did it!" Team members made this statement after they had just finished playing in a community sports tournament. They didn't win the tournament, but they got the team together, entered the tournament, and played several games. They developed a team **strategy** (an overall team plan) and **tactics** (specific methods to reach the team goal) that are necessary to work together as a team.

Being part of a team that works together and supports each other is a lot of fun. Maybe you've already experienced this, but if not, look for the opportunity. Sometimes teamwork brings the thrill of victory when your team wins. But you don't have to win to experience the fun of being part of a team that works hard together, pursues a goal, and does its best.

Team members don't all need to have the same abilities and interests. Teams gain strength when different people contribute different things. You've learned about physical flexibility in this chapter, but that's not the only type of flexibility. Flexibility also means the ability to change. Being able to adapt to different situations is an important part of teamwork.

Use the worksheet supplied by your teacher to develop a strategy for being active with people on your support team. Build good teamwork by giving each person a special role in the group.

Lesson Review

▶ What is flexibility?

▶ How do you build flexibility?

▶ Describe some guidelines for feeling comfortable in physical activity.

▶ How much stretching is enough?

6.2

Benefits of Flexibility

Lesson Vocabulary

cramp, flexion, hypermobility, joint, muscles, range of motion

Click Student Info ▶ Topic 6.6

When you do flexibility exercises, you get health, wellness, and fitness benefits. Can you describe some of the benefits of stretching and good flexibility? Do you have good flexibility? How can you tell whether you have good flexibility? When you finish this lesson, you'll know the answers to these questions. You'll also understand the importance of range of motion to your performance in physical activity.

What Are the Benefits of Flexibility?

There are many benefits to being flexible, including good health, good posture, reduced risk of injury, and improved performance. One of the health benefits of good flexibility is the prevention of back pain. Back pain is a major cause of missed work and results in millions of dollars in medical expenses each year. As many as 80 percent of American adults will experience back pain at some time in their lives. But back pain isn't just a problem for adults. Nearly one third of preteen children have experienced some type of back pain, and the incidence of back problems among teens is nearly as high as for adults. Having good muscle fitness and flexibility in the back, chest, shoulder, neck, and upper leg muscles can reduce the risk of back problems.

Click Student Info ▶ Topic 6.7

Poor flexibility can also contribute to poor posture. Short muscles in the chest can lead to rounded shoulders and can cause the head to lean forward. Short muscles in the back and the back of the leg can cause a curve in the lower back that can result in muscle soreness and pain. Regular stretching can help you maintain good posture.

If a muscle is too short, it's at risk of injury. Frequently injured muscles include the hamstrings (the back of the upper leg), the calf (the back of the lower leg), the quadriceps (the front of the upper leg), and the muscles of the lower back. Regular stretching can lengthen these muscles and reduce the risk of injury. Also, these muscles may **cramp** during exercise. Statically stretching a muscle that has a cramp can cause the cramp to go away. For example, the calf stretch in lesson 6.1 can be used to stop a cramp in the calf muscle.

Good flexibility can also enhance performance in sports and in daily life. A gymnast or a diver must have good flexibility to perform well. The same is true for skateboarding and playing hacky sack. Without good flexibility, you can't perform at your best. Good flexibility is also necessary to perform tasks in your daily life. For example, a person with

> **FIT FACT**
>
> Muscle cramps are often caused by dehydration (not drinking enough water). Replacing water lost when you sweat can help prevent cramps.

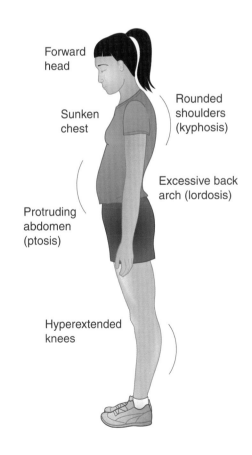

Poor flexibility can contribute to poor posture.

poor range of motion in his neck would have difficulty backing up in a car because he couldn't turn around well. A person with short hamstring muscles would have a hard time bending over to pick up an object from the ground or tie her shoe.

How Do I Know if I Have Good Flexibility?

To be healthy and to perform effectively, you need good flexibility and full range of motion in all joints. There are many tests of flexibility for many parts of the body. The back-saver sit-and-reach is one of the most common tests and is included in Fitnessgram (see table 6.3). This test assesses hip and back flexibility. The scoring for the back-saver sit-and-reach test is different from that of other fitness tests. If you meet the healthy fitness score for your age and gender, you pass the test. To pass the test and have a score in the healthy fitness zone, you must have long muscles in the back of your legs and in your back. Because you might have good flexibility on one side of your body and not on the other, you must do the back-saver sit-and-reach test on both sides.

The Back-Saver Sit-and-Reach Test of Flexibility

The back-saver sit-and-reach test measures the flexibility of your lower back and the muscles on the back of your thigh (hamstrings). As you take the test, use the worksheet supplied by your teacher to record your results and answer the questions about stretching.

1. Place a measuring stick such as a yardstick on top of a 12-inch-high (31 centimeters) box. Have the stick extend 9 inches (23 centimeters) over the box with the lower numbers toward you.

2. To measure flexibility of your right leg, fully extend it and place your right foot flat against the box. Bend your left leg with the knee turned out and your left foot 2 to 3 inches (5 to 8 centimeters) to the side of your straight right leg.

3. Extend your arms forward over the measuring stick. Place your hands on the stick, one on top of the other, with the palms facing down. The middle fingers should be together with the tips of one finger exactly on top of the other.

4. Lean forward and reach with the arms and fingers four times. On the fourth reach, hold the position for 3 seconds and observe the inch mark below your fingertips. Then record your score to the nearest inch.

5. Repeat the test with the left leg straight. Consult table 6.3 to see if you're in the healthy fitness zone, and write the results on your worksheet.

Note: Warm up before performing this test.

Reprinted, by permission, from C. Corbin and R. Lindsey, 2005, *Fitness for life*, 5th ed. (Champaign, IL: Human Kinetics), 82.

Table 6.3

Healthy Fitness Zone for Flexibility (Back-Saver Sit-and-Reach)

Age	Needs improvement	Healthy fitness (pass)
MALES		
10	Less than 8 inches	8 inches
11	Less than 8 inches	8 inches
12	Less than 8 inches	8 inches
13	Less than 8 inches	8 inches
14	Less than 8 inches	8 inches
15+	Less than 8 inches	8 inches
FEMALES		
10	Less than 9 inches	9 inches
11	Less than 10 inches	10 inches
12	Less than 10 inches	10 inches
13	Less than 10 inches	10 inches
14	Less than 10 inches	10 inches
15+	Less than 12 inches	12 inches

8 inches = 20 centimeters; 9 inches = 23 centimeters; 10 inches = 25 centimeters; 12 inches = 31 centimeters

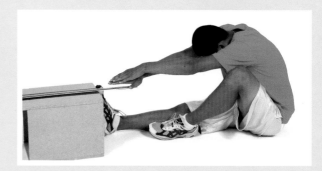

Biomechanical Principles: Range of Motion

Your body joints allow a certain amount of motion in each possible direction, and exceeding that limit can cause injury.

A **joint** is the location where your bones (your body's levers) join together. Each joint allows motion in certain directions, and in each direction there is a range of motion. The amount of movement that a joint allows is called **range of motion.** Some joints allow movement in more directions than others. For example, the hip joint is where the bones of the pelvis join with the bones of the thigh. The hip joint allows forward and backward movement (see photo below left). The thigh can also be moved to the side or rotated (moved in a circle) around the hip joint. The upper arm can be moved in similar ways around the shoulder joint (see photo below right).

The knees and elbows have more limited directions of motion (see the photos on page 74). They can flex and extend, but they don't bend sideways or twist. In other words, these joints have no range of motion in certain directions. You should know how much range of motion a joint will allow when doing flexibility and muscle fitness exercises. Forcing a joint to move beyond a safe range of motion in any direction can result in injury to ligaments, tendons, and **muscles.** For example, when you do a full squat such as a catcher does in baseball, the weight of the body on the levers of your legs can

cause your knee to bend too much. Doing an exercise such as a full squat with weight on your shoulders is bad because it can cause injury to the knee.

If you know about the normal range of motion of your joints, you can avoid exercises and movements that can cause injury. Stretching to increase flexibility can increase range of motion by lengthening tendons and muscles. However, stretching beyond the normal range of motion is dangerous, because it can leave a joint too loose to provide needed stability for the body. **Hypermobility** is a term used to describe joints that lack stability and have too much range of motion. When stretching to increase flexibility, don't force joints to move in directions where they have no range of motion. For instance, twisting or bending sideways at the knee can cause damage to the knee ligaments, which hold the joint together.

Applying the Principle

As you learned earlier, each joint has its own range of motion in each possible direction. Movements that cause a joint to move beyond its normal range of motion in a particular direction can cause small injuries in the joint that can lead to bigger injuries later in life. An example of movements that cause too much range of motion in joints is too much bending (**flexion**) of the

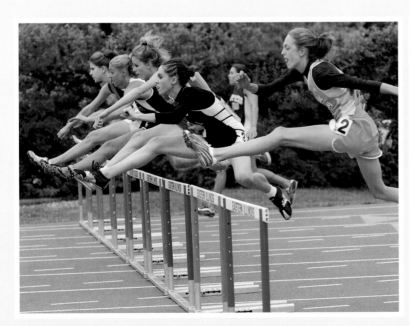

Running hurdles requires good range of motion in the hips.

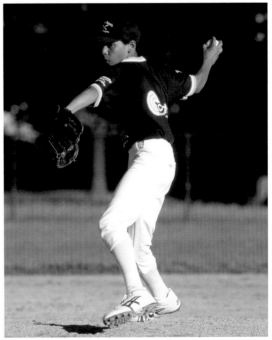

Pitching in baseball requires good range of motion in the shoulders.

(continued)

Biomechanical Principles: Range of Motion   *(continued)*

knee by a catcher in baseball. That's why catchers wear special pads on the backs of their legs to stop them from doing a full squat. It's also dangerous to bend the knee to the side, bend too far forward while standing (as in the standing toe touch), or bend too far backward (as in the back arch exercise).

In which direction(s) is it appropriate to move each of these joints? In which direction(s) is it not appropriate? Describe an activity that uses each of these joints in the best range of motion.

▶ Hip
▶ Shoulder
▶ Knee
▶ Elbow

Principles in Practice

It's important to know how to move joints through a normal range of motion to prevent injury. Move each of the following joints through its comfortable range of motion in each direction to determine your current range of motion: shoulders, elbows, wrists, hips, knees, ankles, and neck. Do you have the same range of motion on both sides of your body?

Always avoid exercises and activities that require unsafe ranges of motion, and practice only the exercises that have a safe range of motion. All of the exercises in this book have a safe range of motion except those that are shown to describe unsafe exercises. The purpose of exercise is to improve your ability to move, not to damage your joints, muscles, or bones.

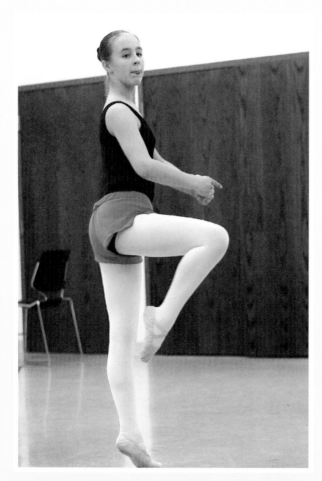

The hip allows motion in several directions, while the knee only allows motion in flexion or extension.

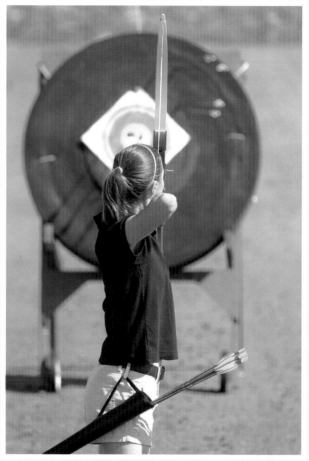

The elbow only allows flexion and extension, while the shoulder allows motion in several directions.

Click Student Info ▶ Topic 6.8

You can have flexibility in one part of the body and not have it in another. The back-saver sit-and-reach test assesses range of motion in the lower body. The shoulder stretch test assesses shoulder flexibility and is sometimes included in Fitnessgram. You can learn more about this test and other flexibility assessments by visiting the *Fitness for Life: Middle School* Web site.

Click Student Info ▶ Topic 6.9

Once you've taken a flexibility test, you'll need to determine if your score is in the healthy fitness zone. Use table 6.3 on page 72 to see if you're in the healthy fitness zone for the back-saver sit-and-reach test. If you fall below the healthy fitness zone, you should improve your flexibility. If you're in the healthy fitness zone, you might want to do regular stretching exercises to become even more flexible. Scores above the healthy

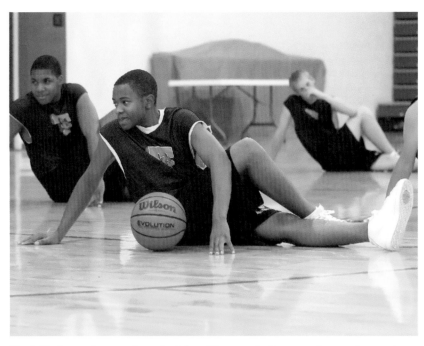

Stretching exercises are important for all teens, whether you play sports or not.

fitness zone may be beneficial to those interested in athletic and specific types of performance, but they're not necessary to achieve the other benefits described earlier in this chapter. In some cases, too much stretching or too much flexibility can increase the chance of injury (see Biomechanical Principles on pages 73-74).

Stretching exercises are an important part of a complete physical activity program for teens. When performed regularly, stretching exercises build flexibility that provides the benefits described in this chapter.

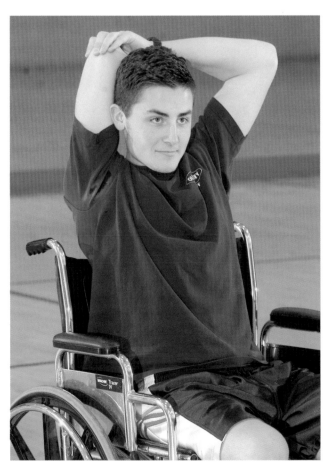

Even if you're already in the healthy fitness zone, regular stretching exercises can help you become more flexible.

Lesson Review

▶ How does good flexibility improve your health, wellness, and fitness?

▶ How do you know if you have good flexibility?

▶ How is range of motion important to performance in physical activity?

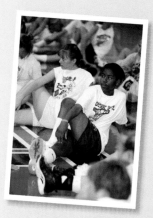

6 Chapter Review

Number your paper from 1 to 5. Read each question. After the number for the question, write a word or a phrase that best answers the question. The page number where you can find the answer is listed after the question.

1. What term describes the amount of movement in a joint? (page 65)
2. What word describes tissue that connects bone to bone? (page 66)
3. What is another word used in this chapter to describe static or nonmoving? (page 66)
4. How many seconds should you hold each static stretch of a muscle to get the best benefits? (page 70)
5. What health problem associated with poor flexibility occurs in 80 percent of adults at some time in their lives? (page 71)

Number your paper from 6 to 10. Next to each number, write the letter of the best answer.

6. gravity   a. one aid in producing a static stretch
7. tendon   b. an injury to a muscle
8. back-saver sit-and-reach   c. tissue that connects muscle to bone
9. strain   d. a test of flexibility
10. hypermobility   e. too much range of motion

Number your paper from 11 to 15. Follow the directions to answer each question or statement.

11. Explain the difference between a static stretch and PNF stretch.
12. Give three or more examples of static stretching exercises for building flexibility.
13. Give three or more examples of guidelines for feeling more comfortable in physical activity.
14. Give three or more examples of the health benefits of good flexibility.
15. Give examples of the normal range of motion for two different joints.

Ask the Authors

When is the best time to do stretching exercises to improve flexibility?
    Get the answer and ask your own questions at the *Fitness for Life: Middle School* Web site.

Click Student Info ▶ Topic 6.10

Unit Review on the Web

You can find unit II review materials on the *Fitness for Life: Middle School* Web site.

Click Student Info ▶ Topic 6.11

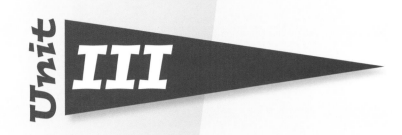

Unit III

Muscle Fitness, Body Composition, and Planning

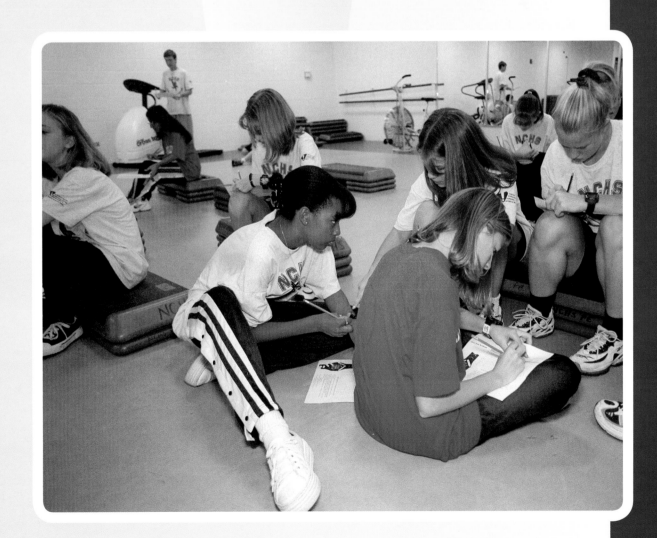

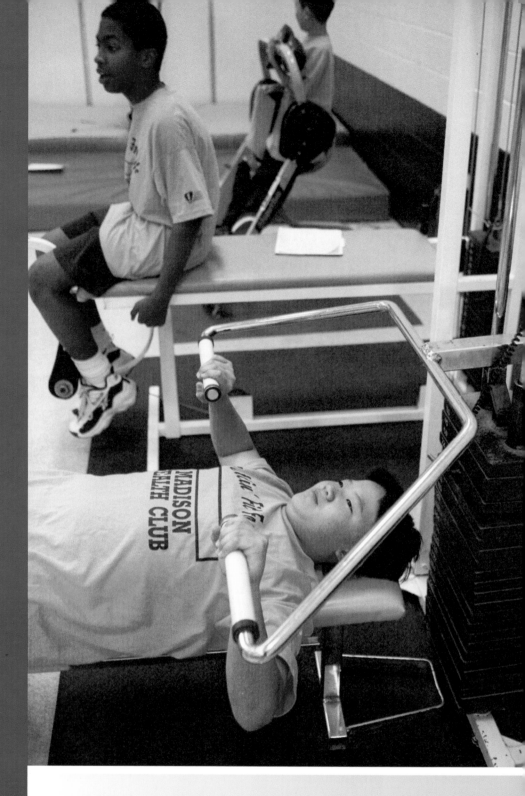

7

Muscle Fitness Exercises

In this chapter...

Muscle Fitness Exercises: Level 3 of the Physical Activity Pyramid

Lesson Vocabulary

isometric exercises, isotonic exercise, muscle fitness, principle of overload, principle of progression, progressive resistance exercise (PRE), repetition (rep), set, supplements

▶ **www.fitnessforlife.org/middleschool/**
Click Student Info ▶ Topic 7.1

One of the types of activities in the Physical Activity Pyramid is muscle fitness exercise. Do you know what muscle fitness is? Do you know the best way to safely build muscle fitness? Do you need supplements to build muscle fitness? When you finish this lesson, you'll know the answers to these questions. You'll also become aware of some guidelines for preventing bullying in physical activity settings.

What Is Muscle Fitness?

There are two parts of **muscle fitness:** muscular strength and muscular endurance. Strength is the amount of force a muscle can exert. Lifting a weight such as a heavy bag of groceries is an example of using strength. Muscular endurance is the ability to use the muscles for long periods of time without getting tired. Carrying a grocery bag from the store to your home is an example of using muscular endurance. You need both strength and muscular endurance to have good muscle fitness.

Strength and muscular endurance are similar, but they're not the same thing. A strong person typically has bigger muscles than a person who isn't as strong. People who have good muscular endurance don't necessarily have big muscles, but their muscle fibers don't tire as easily. A person who is strong enough to lift a heavy weight might not be able to lift a lighter weight as many times as a person with higher muscular endurance could. On the other hand, a person with good muscular endurance might not be able to lift as much weight as a person who has greater strength.

How Do I Build Muscle Fitness?

To build muscle fitness, you must follow the **principle of overload.** This principle says that you must make your muscles work more than they normally do if you want to improve muscle fitness. Milo of Crotona, a Greek wrestler and soldier who lived nearly 3,000 years ago, used overload to become one of the strongest men in the world. When he was a boy, he lifted a calf. As Milo grew, so did the calf. Milo became stronger and stronger as he lifted the calf, which became heavier and heavier. Lifting more and more weight caused an overload on Milo's muscles and helped make him strong and fit. Like Milo, you must overload your muscles if you want to build muscle fitness.

Many kinds of exercises build muscle fitness by overloading your muscles. For example, you can lift weights or use an exercise resistance machine. These exercises are called resistance exercises because they cause your muscles to overcome resistance. Sometimes the term *progressive resistance exercise (PRE)* is used.

Milo used the principle of overload to build muscle fitness.

This is because one of the principles of muscle fitness is the **principle of progression**. This principle says that you should increase resistance progressively (little by little) when exercising to build muscle fitness. The example of Milo and the calf illustrates the importance of progression. As the calf grew older and older and gained weight, the amount of weight Milo lifted gradually increased. Progressive overload allows the muscles to improve gradually. For beginners, too much too soon can cause soreness, fatigue, and even injury. Even for a person who does regular PRE, there are limits to what can be achieved. For example, Milo would not have been able to lift a fully grown bull that weighed 1,000 pounds (450 kilograms) or more. So we all need to follow a program that is reasonable. Progressive resistance exercises for building muscle fitness are included at the third level of the Physical Activity Pyramid.

What Are Some Types of Progressive Resistance Exercise?

The most common type of resistance exercise for building muscle fitness is **isotonic exercise.** When you do isotonic exercises, you contract your muscles to produce movement. Examples of isotonic exercises include weight training (dumbbells and barbells), using resistance exercise machines, using exercise bands, and performing calisthenics such as push-ups and sit-ups. Visit the *Fitness for Life: Middle School* Web site to learn more about isotonic and other exercises.

Click Student Info ← Topic 7.2

When you do resistance exercises in which there is no movement, you're doing **isometric exercises.** When you do this type of exercise, your muscles still contract to exert force, but they work against an immovable object. For example, you can push your hands against each other as hard as you can or pull against a towel.

Table 7.1 shows examples of isometric and isotonic exercises.

How Do I Exercise Safely?

In the past, people believed that resistance training was dangerous for children and teens. Experts now know that resistance training to build muscle fitness can be safe for young people if done properly. Some guidelines that middle school students should follow for doing resistance training safely are listed below. Different guidelines for older teens and adults are available at the *Fitness for Life: Middle School* Web site.

- Use proper technique. Before doing an exercise, learn to do it properly.
- Consult with an expert (such as your physical education teacher) before beginning.
- Consider calisthenics that use your body weight to build muscle fitness.
- Use moderate resistance. Young teens shouldn't use maximal resistance for isotonic exercises (see table 7.2).
- Use the "three S" method for isotonic exercises—movements should be slow, smooth, and steady.
- Breathe when exercising. Don't hold your breath when doing resistance exercises.
- Use a spotter, especially for weight training with barbells and dumbbells. A spotter is a person who stands near the lifter to make sure that the weight does not fall on the lifter.
- Avoid competition in resistance training.

Click Student Info ← Topic 7.3

Level 3

Rest or inactivity

Exercise for strength and muscular endurance

F = 2-3 days a week
I = Moderate resistance
T = 10 to 25 reps, 1 to 3 sets

Exercise for flexibility

Active aerobics

Active sports and recreation

Lifestyle physical activity

Strength and muscular endurance exercises are at level 3 of the Physical Activity Pyramid.

Table 7.1

Types of Progressive Resistance Exercises

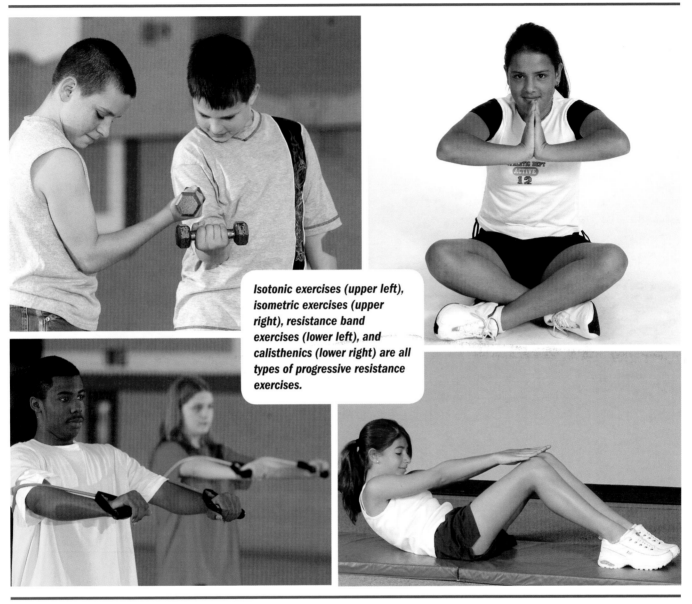

Isotonic exercises (upper left), isometric exercises (upper right), resistance band exercises (lower left), and calisthenics (lower right) are all types of progressive resistance exercises.

Table 7.2

FIT Formula for Muscle Fitness for Teens

	Strength	Muscular endurance
ISOTONIC EXERCISE		
Frequency	Two to three days a week (nonconsecutive days)	Three to six days a week
Intensity	Moderate resistance exercises that you can do 15 times or fewer (if you can do more than 15 reps, the resistance is too low)	Low resistance exercises that you can do at least 25 times (25 reps)
Time	One set of 10 to 15 reps	One to three sets of 11 to 25 reps
ISOMETRIC EXERCISE		
Frequency	Two or three days a week (nonconsecutive days)	Three to six days a week
Intensity	Contract as tightly as possible.	Moderate contractions
Time	Contract the muscle for 7 to 10 seconds; do one to three reps.	Contract the muscle for 11 to 25 seconds; do one to three reps.

How Much Exercise Do I Need to Build Muscle Fitness?

To overload your muscles, you must repeat resistance exercises several times. Each time you perform an exercise, you complete a **repetition.** If you do an exercise 10 times in a row, you've done 10 repetitions. Sometimes the word *rep* is used as an abbreviation of the word *repetition.* A group of several reps of an exercise is called a **set.** You should have a period of rest between sets. (See the upper figure below.)

The FIT formula described in table 7.2 will help you decide how many repetitions and sets you need to do to build muscle fitness. There is a different FIT formula for each of the two types of muscle fitness. There is also a different FIT formula for isotonic and isometric exercises. As table 7.2 indicates, you use more resistance and fewer reps to build strength, and you use less resistance and more reps to build muscular endurance. For example, if you were lifting weights, you would lift heavier weights fewer times to build strength, and you would lift lighter weights more times to build muscular endurance. (See the lower figure below.)

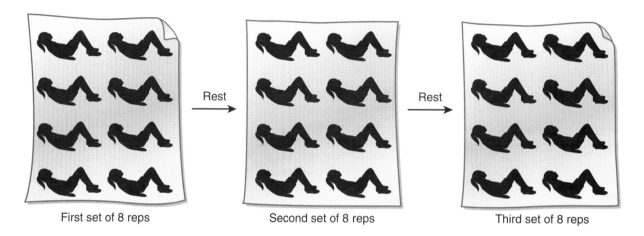

First set of 8 reps   Second set of 8 reps   Third set of 8 reps

Progressive resistance exercises for muscle fitness require you to do reps and sets.

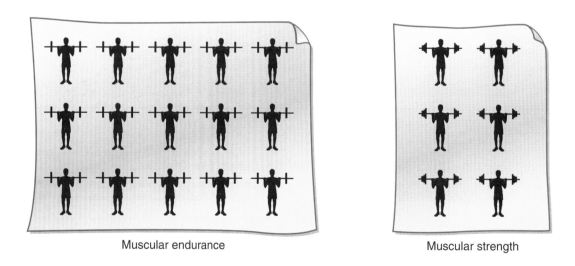

Muscular endurance   Muscular strength

Muscular endurance requires more reps and less weight, while muscular strength requires more weight and fewer reps.

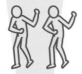

Moving Together:
Bullying

Have you or someone you know ever been bullied? How did you feel about it? What did you do about it? Why do you think some students are bullies? How can you help prevent bullying?

Dominique is shorter than other kids in his class. His dad says he is a late developer. He told Dominique not to worry because he would start to grow soon. But Dominique wants to grow now. Sometimes other kids tease him in the locker room. A couple of kids really pick on him and send him mean e-mail messages. His friend Greg helps him avoid the bullies, but Greg isn't always around when Dominique needs him. Dominique doesn't tell his teacher or his parents that he's being bullied because he doesn't want to seem weak. He's also afraid that if the bullies find out he told, they might bully him even more.

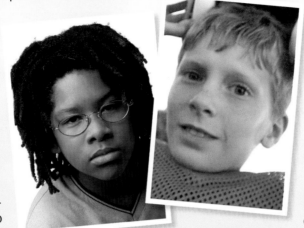

Discussion Questions

1. What can Dominique do to avoid problems in the locker room and in other places?

2. What can Dominique do to improve his muscle fitness both in the short term and the long term?

3. What keeps other kids from helping Dominique with his problem?

4. How can Greg be of more help to Dominique than he already is?

5. Do you think Dominique's mom and dad can help him?

Guidelines for Preventing Bullying

▶ *Learn about bullies and why they bully.* Bullies are people who try to intimidate others to gain attention and to feel important. The more attention they get for their behavior, the more likely they are to repeat it.

▶ *Recognize that people who are bullied are not the problem.* A teen who is bullied rarely is the cause of the problem. Bullies are the problem. The person who is bullied should not feel guilty, and people who see bullying shouldn't believe that it is the victim's fault. Bullying can happen to anyone.

▶ *Check to see if your school has rules concerning bullying.* Bullying is an antisocial behavior that schools want to prevent. In recent years many schools have developed guidelines to prevent bullying, including cyberbullying (sending mean e-mails and text messages). Find out if your school has guidelines for preventing bullying.

▶ *Collective action is better than action by one person.* Sometimes it's best to get help from others when dealing with a problem such as bullying, including cyberbullying (sending mean e-mails and text messages). The next three guidelines provide information on getting help from others.

▶ *Communicate with your parents or guardians.* People who are picked on or bullied sometimes don't want to tell their parents or loved ones. They may think that this makes them look weak. They also may worry that their parents will do something that will cause them more problems. Having open communication with your parents or guardians on a regular basis can help make things easier when a problem exists. If you're being bullied, speak honestly about it to your parent or guardian.

▶ *Communicate with your teacher or guidance counselor.* If you're being bullied, you may want to have a parent or guardian with you when you talk to school officials about the bullying. Talks with school officials may help you find out about school policy and the best way to make sure the policy is enforced.

▶ *Communicate with your friends.* When bullies see that others don't support their behavior, they are less likely to bully someone. Bullies usually try to find situations in which they have the support of their own friends and the victim is alone or has little support from friends. Talk to your friends about bullies and come to the support of others when necessary.

▶ *Plan a strategy.* Try to avoid situations in which a bully has an advantage, such as when you're alone, when a teacher isn't available to witness the problem or provide help, and when the bully has the support of other bullies.

Become part of the solution by signing the Respect and Protect Oath supplied by your teacher.

Click Student Info ▶ **Topic 7.4**

Do I Need Supplements?

Teens who want to build muscle fitness sometimes want fast results. They may think that the answer is to take **supplements** with long names that promise to build fitness and increase performance. The Food and Drug Administration (FDA), a government agency that regulates foods and drugs, defines a supplement as "a product taken by mouth that contains a 'dietary ingredient' intended to supplement the diet." Supplements are different from medicines. Medicines must be approved by the FDA before they can be sold, but the FDA doesn't have to test and approve supplements. Supplements include vitamins, minerals, herbs, proteins, and many other substances. They're found in many forms such as tablets, capsules, gelcaps, liquids, or powders and bars that look similar to candy bars.

Eating good food and performing regular muscle fitness exercise is the best way to build muscle fitness. Supplements are costly and unnecessary, and they might contain substances other than what are listed on the package. Because supplements aren't regulated by the government, there's no guarantee that you're getting what you think you're getting when you buy a supplement. You should also know that supplements can cause side effects or unwanted negative problems including headaches, dehydration, changes in heartbeat, and allergies. The people who advertise supplements rarely warn you of the side effects. You should consider supplements only when your doctor has recommended them and your parent or guardian approves.

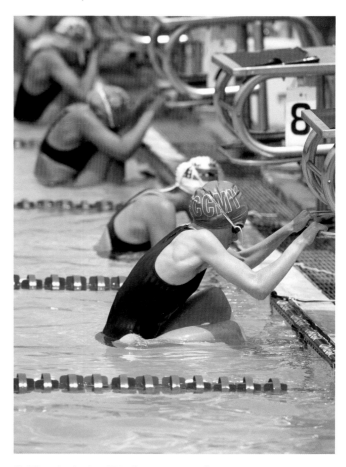

Holding the body still before the start of a race requires isometric strength.

Take It Home

Building Muscle and Character

Strength can be displayed in many ways. Physical strength is needed for rock climbing and cheerleading. In this chapter you learned how to build muscles to improve physical strength. Mental strength is tested during a chess match. You learn how to improve mental strength in many of the classes you take in school.

Strength of character is another kind of strength. It's tested daily, and it defines you as a person. Are you honest? Do you play fair? Do you take responsibility for your own actions? Do you stand up for others even when it's the unpopular thing to do? Do you respect others regardless of their age, gender, and ethnic background? Are you a caring person? Are you a good citizen in your class, neighborhood, community, and country? Your answers to these and other questions indicate your strength of character.

Use the worksheet supplied by your teacher to show how you can demonstrate strength of character in physical education.

Lesson Review

▶ What is muscle fitness?

▶ Describe the overload principle and the principle of progression, and explain how they're important to muscle fitness development.

▶ Define the terms isotonic exercise and isometric exercise, and give examples of each type of exercise.

▶ Describe the FIT formulas for building strength and muscular endurance.

▶ Describe several guidelines for performing muscle fitness exercises safely.

▶ Do you need supplements to build muscle fitness?

▶ Describe some guidelines for preventing bullying in physical activity settings.

Benefits of Muscle Fitness Exercises

Lesson Vocabulary
gravity, osteoporosis, resistance, specificity

Click Student Info ▶ Topic 7.5

When you do muscle fitness exercises, you gain health, wellness, and fitness benefits. Can you describe some of the benefits of muscle fitness? Do you have good muscle fitness? How can you tell? Do you know what things other than activity affect your muscle fitness? When you finish this lesson, you'll know the answers to these questions. You'll also understand the importance of resistance to your performance in physical activity.

What Are the Benefits of Muscle Fitness?

There are many benefits of muscle fitness. As with flexibility, the benefits include good health, good posture, a reduced risk of injury, and improved performance. Good muscle fitness can also help you feel and look your best.

One of the major health benefits of having good muscle fitness is strong, healthy bones. **Osteoporosis** is a disease that occurs when the bones become weak. Regular progressive resistance exercises help build strong bones and help reduce the risk of osteoporosis. Also, performing muscle fitness exercises regularly has been associated with good cardiovascular health including healthy blood pressure and healthy levels of fat in the blood.

The combination of good muscle fitness and good flexibility (see chapter 6) is especially important for good posture and good back health. Good muscle fitness and flexibility also help reduce the risk of muscle strains that can occur in sports and active jobs. For example, muscular endurance is important for soccer and hockey, and strength is important in wrestling, gymnastics, football, and track and field events such as putting the shot and throwing the discus. Wildlife photographers, news crews, letter carriers, construction workers, and people in many other occupations need to have good muscle fitness to do their jobs.

Strong muscles can also help prevent injuries to joints such as the knees and ankles by building muscles to support them. Good muscle fitness can also help you to get well after an injury. People who have injured an ankle, a knee, or another body part can benefit from progressive resistance training.

Click Student Info ▶ Topic 7.6

Muscle fitness can help you control body weight and look your best. Having strong muscles in the abdominal region can help keep your abdomen from sticking out. Good muscle fitness helps you maintain a good posture as well. Also, people with well-developed muscles burn more calories than people with less developed muscles. This is true even when they're not doing exercise. For this reason a person with

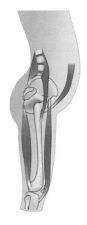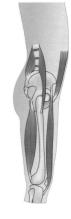

The person on the left has an excessive low back curve and protruding abdomen because of weak muscles. The person on the right has good posture (healthy low back curve and flat abdomen) because of strong muscles.

good muscle fitness is more likely to avoid gaining excess fat than a person with poor muscle fitness. Together, these factors can help you look your best. Good muscle fitness also helps you to feel good because if you're fit, you can perform daily activities and leisure activities without undue fatigue.

Click Student Info ▶ Topic 7.7

How Much Muscle Fitness Is Enough?

Muscle fitness is important for everyone. But we don't all need the same amount. Experts agree that you should have at least enough muscle fitness to score in the healthy fitness zone if you want to gain the health benefits described earlier in this chapter. To determine your muscle fitness, you'll take three different tests from Fitnessgram: the push-up test (below), the curl-up test (page 87), and the trunk

lift test (page 87). You can learn to perform these tests by yourself so that you can keep track of your improvements. The curl-up, push-up, and trunk lift tests measure both strength and muscular endurance. The trunk lift test requires good flexibility as well as good muscle fitness.

You can use tables 7.3 (males) or 7.4 (females) to see if you're in the healthy fitness zone for each test. If your score falls below the healthy fitness zone, you'll want to do progressive resistance exercises that will help you improve. If you're in the healthy fitness zone, you'll want to do regular progressive resistance exercises to maintain that level or to move to a higher level within the zone. Many teens do progressive resistance exercises to build muscle fitness for special purposes such as preparing for a sport, preparing for a ski trip or a dance recital, preparing for a job, or feeling and looking their best. You can consult with your teacher about the best way to meet your muscle fitness goals.

Push-Up Test

1. Lie facedown on a mat or carpet with your hands under your shoulders, your fingers spread, and your legs straight. Your legs should be slightly apart and your toes should be tucked under.

2. Push up until your arms are straight. Keep your legs and back straight. Your body should form a straight line.

3. Lower your body by bending your elbows until your upper arms are parallel to the floor (at a 90-degree angle), then push up until the arms are fully extended. Do one push-up every 3 seconds. You may want to have a partner say "up-down" every 3 seconds to help you. You're finished when you fail to complete a push-up with proper form for the second time.

   If you have not done push-ups in a while, you may want to stop at 15 (for females) or 25 (for males) because these scores put you well into the healthy fitness zone no matter what your age. Doing too much too soon can

result in soreness. When you have performed push-ups regularly for a while, you may want to try to increase scores within the healthy fitness zone.

4. Record the number of push-ups you performed on your worksheet. Then find your rating in table 7.3 or 7.4 on page 88.

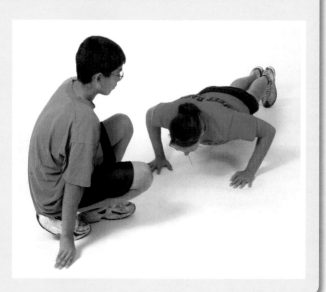

Adapted, by permission, from C. Corbin and R. Lindsey, 2005, *Fitness for life*, 5th ed. (Champaign, IL: Human Kinetics), 30-31.

Curl-Up Test

1. Lie on your back on a mat or a carpet. Bend your knees approximately 140 degrees. Your feet should be slightly apart and flat on the floor. Your arms should be straight and parallel to your trunk with the palms of the hands resting on the mat. Make sure you have extended your feet as far as possible from the buttocks while still allowing the feet to remain flat on the floor. The closer your feet are positioned in relation to the buttocks, the more difficult the movement.

2. Place your head on a piece of paper. The paper will assist your partner in judging if your head touched down on each repetition. Place a 4 1/2 inch strip (11 centimeters; cardboard, rubber, or plastic) under your knees so that the fingers of both hands just touch the near edge of the strip. A partner can stand on the strip to keep it stationary or you can tape it down.

3. Keeping your heels on the floor, curl your shoulders up slowly and slide your arms forward so that the fingers move across the cardboard strip. Curl up until the fingertips reach the far side of the strip.

4. Slowly lower your back until your head rests on the piece of paper.

Adapted, by permission, from C. Corbin and R. Lindsey, 2005, *Fitness for life, 5th ed.* (Champaign, IL: Human Kinetics), 29.

5. Repeat the procedure so that you do one curl-up every 3 seconds. A partner could help you by saying "up-down" every 3 seconds. You're finished when you can't do another curl up or when you fail to keep up with the 3-second count.

   If you have not done curl-ups in a while, you may want to stop at 25 because this score puts you well into the healthy fitness zone no matter what your age. Doing too much too soon can result in soreness. When you have performed curl-ups regularly for a while, you may want to try to increase scores within the healthy fitness zone.

6. Record the number of curl-ups you have completed on your worksheet. Then find your rating in table 7.3 or 7.4 on page 88.

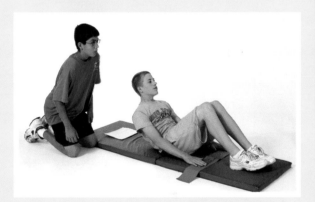

Trunk Lift Test

1. Lie facedown with your arms to your sides and your hands under your thighs.

2. Lift the upper part of your body very slowly so that your chin, chest, and shoulders come off the floor. Lift your trunk as high as possible to a maximum of 12 inches (31 centimeters). Hold this position while a partner measures the distance your chin lifts off the floor (about 3 seconds to allow measurement). The ruler should be at least 1 inch (2 centimeters) in front of your chin. Look straight ahead (at a coin on the mat, for example) to avoid tipping the chin upward.

   Caution: Your partner should not place the ruler directly under your chin in case you have to lower your trunk unexpectedly.

Adapted, by permission, from C. Corbin and R. Lindsey, 2005, *Fitness for life, 5th ed.* (Champaign, IL: Human Kinetics), 122.

3. Do the trunk lift two times and record the number of inches you can lift and hold your chin. Do not record scores above 12 inches (31 centimeters). Use table 7.3 or 7.4 on page 88 to determine your fitness rating. Record your results on your worksheet.

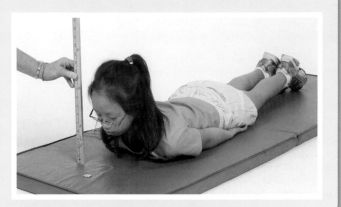

Table 7.3

Muscle Fitness Ratings for Males

Age	Needs improvement	Healthy fitness zone
CURL-UPS (MEASURED IN REPS)		
10	0–11	12–24
11	0–14	15–28
12	0–17	18–36
13	0–20	21–40
14	0–23	24–45
15+	0–23	24–47
PUSH-UPS (MEASURED IN REPS)		
10	0–6	7–20
11	0–7	8–20
12	0–9	10–20
13	0–11	12–25
14	0–13	14–30
15+	0–15	16–35
TRUNK LIFT (MEASURED IN INCHES)*		
10	Less than 9	9–12
11	Less than 9	9–12
12	Less than 9	9–12
13	Less than 9	9–12
14	Less than 9	9–12
15+	Less than 9	9–12

9 inches = 23 centimeters; 12 inches = 31 centimeters

*Must hold above 9 inches (23 centimeters) long enough to allow measurement.

Data generated from Fitnessgram software.

Table 7.4

Muscle Fitness Ratings for Females

Age	Needs improvement	Healthy fitness zone
CURL-UPS (MEASURED IN REPS)		
10	0–11	12–26
11	0–14	15–29
12	0–17	18–32
13	0–17	18–32
14	0–17	18–32
15+	0–17	18–35
PUSH-UPS (MEASURED IN REPS)		
10	0–6	7–15
11	0–6	7–15
12	0–6	7–15
13	0–6	7–15
14	0–6	7–15
15+	0–6	7–15
TRUNK LIFT (MEASURED IN INCHES)*		
10	Less than 9	9–12
11	Less than 9	9–12
12	Less than 9	9–12
13	Less than 9	9–12
14	Less than 9	9–12
15+	Less than 9	9–12

9 inches = 23 centimeters; 12 inches = 31 centimeters

*Must hold above 9 inches (23 centimeters) long enough to allow measurement.

Data generated from Fitnessgram software.

What Else Affects My Muscle Fitness?

The best way to build muscle fitness is to do regular muscle fitness exercises using the information you learned in this chapter. But you should know that factors other than exercise influence your muscle fitness. These include sex, age, maturation, and heredity. Preteen girls and boys often have similar scores on muscle fitness tests and often do similar activities. By the teen years, boys typically have higher muscle fitness scores than girls because during the teen years male hormones cause boys to build bigger muscles than girls. As boys and girls grow older, they'll score higher on the Fitnessgram tests than they did when they were younger. You'll notice that the scores required to get in the healthy fitness zone are higher for boys than for girls on most tests, and that the scores increase as teens grow older.

Some girls might think that muscle fitness isn't for them because they don't have fitness scores simi-lar to boys. However, research shows that muscle fitness helps girls to feel and look their best and to do daily activities without fatigue. Good muscle fitness also builds the bones and prevents bone problems that are common in women later in life. Muscle also burns many calories and helps you to maintain a healthy body weight.

Teens who mature earlier often score better than those who mature later. Also, some people are born with more fast-twitch muscle fibers than others are. People with more fast-twitch fibers typically can build stronger muscles than those with fewer fast-twitch fibers. Bigger muscles can produce more force than smaller ones can. You also inherit slow-twitch fibers from your parents. People with high numbers of slow-twitch fibers respond well to muscular endurance exercise as well as exercise requiring good cardiovascular fitness. The most important thing is to get into the healthy fitness zone, not how you compare with other people.

Click Student Info ▶ Topic 7.8

Biomechanical Principles:
Resistance

Air, water, gravity, friction, and other external forces provide resistance to human movement.

Force is created when muscles use energy to contract. When muscles contract, they move the body's levers, causing the body to move. **Resistance** is opposition to a force or a movement. Air can cause resistance to body movement and it can cause resistance to an object, such as a ball when it is thrown. This resistance can cause slower movement. For example, you can run faster with the wind than against it. Some Olympic runners wear special suits to reduce air resistance so that they can run faster.

Water provides even more resistance than air. Swimmers learn to move through the water with as little resistance to their body movement as possible. Olympic swimmers wear special swimsuits that cut down the resistance of the water.

Gravity is the force that causes objects to fall toward earth. It causes resistance to movements such as jumping upward. On the moon there is less gravity, so astronauts find less resistance to movement and are able to jump higher than they could on earth.

Lifting a heavy weight is harder than lifting a light weight because gravity pulls down more on the heavy weight. Other external forces can also cause resistance to movement. A football player trying to block another football player has to overcome the resistance of the forward movement of the other player.

Resistance can have a negative effect on certain performances, but it can have a positive effect on others. You already know that air resistance can slow a runner, water resistance can slow a swimmer, and resistance from gravity limits how high you can jump. But resistance can also be used in a positive way. For example, swimmers rely on the resistance of the water against their hands to be able to pull themselves through the water. Also, resistance can be used to overload the muscles and so build muscle fitness. Exercise machines use resistance produced by a machine to overload your muscles. Weights such as dumbbells and barbells also cause resistance that overloads the muscles. In these cases, the resistance is good because it helps you to build muscle fitness.

Applying the Principle

Resistance can make it harder to do a movement, and in some cases it can be used to make a movement easier. In some cases resistance can be used to build the muscles through overload. For each of the following activities, describe how resistance will make the activity harder or easier. In which activities can resistance be used to build the muscles of the body?

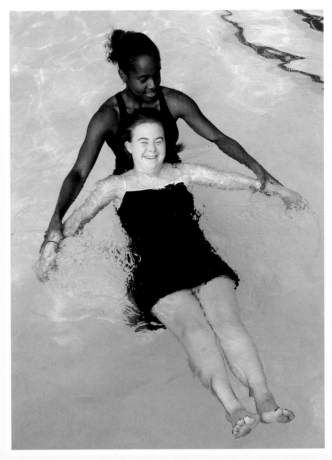

Water provides resistance to movement, but resistance of water against your arms and hands also helps you to move in water.

- ▶ Mowing the lawn
- ▶ Playing tug-of-war
- ▶ Doing push-ups
- ▶ Doing biceps curls
- ▶ Wrestling
- ▶ Playing softball
- ▶ Running with and against the wind
- ▶ Swimming

Principles in Practice

Resistance is important to most physical activities. How can you use resistance to improve performance? What skills can you practice to get better at overcoming resistance? How can you use resistance to build the muscles of the body? What skills can you practice to get better at using resistance to build fitness?

Click Student Info ▶ Topic 7.9

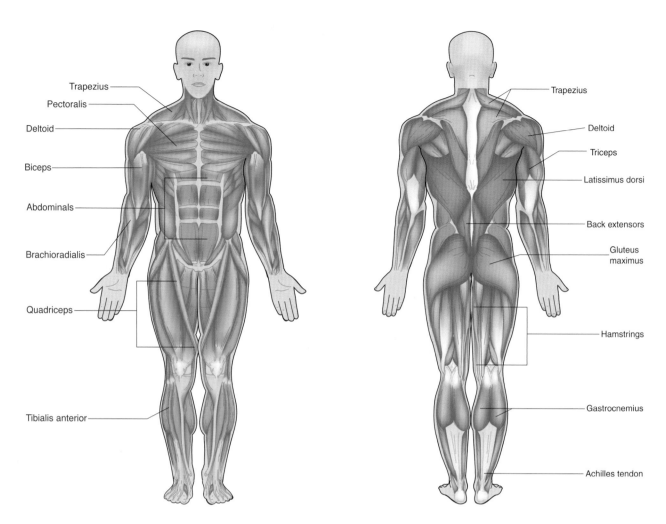

Trapezius
Pectoralis
Deltoid
Biceps
Abdominals
Brachioradialis
Quadriceps
Tibialis anterior

Trapezius
Deltoid
Triceps
Latissimus dorsi
Back extensors
Gluteus maximus
Hamstrings
Gastrocnemius
Achilles tendon

Major muscle groups of the body, front and rear.

Reprinted, by permission, from C. Corbin and R. Lindsey, 2005, *Fitness for life, 5th ed.* (Champaign, IL: Human Kinetics), 151-152.

Which Muscles Should I Exercise?

To get the most from muscle fitness exercises, you should follow the principle of **specificity**. This principle states that to build specific muscles, you must perform exercises for those specific muscles. The illustrations above show the major muscle groups. Labels appear on the muscles that are most important for good health and for successful performance in daily living and in sports and games. You can learn more about the specific types of exercises for building each of these muscles by visiting the *Fitness for Life: Middle School* Web site.

Click Student Info ▶ Topic 7.10

Lesson Review

- ▶ Describe several of the benefits of having good muscle fitness.
- ▶ Describe several of the tests that can be used to assess muscle fitness.
- ▶ Describe the principle of specificity, and explain why it's important to muscle fitness.
- ▶ What factors other than activity affect muscle fitness?
- ▶ How is resistance important to performance in physical activity?

7

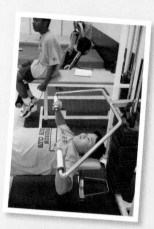

Chapter Review

Number your paper from 1 to 5. Read each question. After the number for the question, write a word or a phrase that best answers the question. The page number where you can find the answer is listed after the question.

1. What principle does the story of Milo illustrate? (page 79)
2. What principle states that you should increase resistance gradually to build muscle fitness? (page 80)
3. What word describes muscle fitness exercises that use your own body weight as resistance? (page 80)
4. What word describes pills that some people take because they think it will improve their muscle fitness? (page 84)
5. What principle states that the benefits from exercise depend on the exercise that you perform? (page 90)

Number your paper from 6 to 10. Next to each number, write the letter of the best answer.

6. reps   **a.** exercises that don't involve movement
7. set   **b.** good for muscular endurance
8. isotonic   **c.** a group of repetitions
9. isometric   **d.** the number of times you do an exercise
10. slow-twitch fibers   **e.** exercises that involve movement

Number your paper from 11 to 15. Follow the directions to answer each question or statement.

11. Explain the difference between strength and muscular endurance.
12. Give several examples of guidelines for performing resistance exercises safely.
13. Give several examples of guidelines for preventing bullying.
14. Name the three Fitnessgram tests of muscle fitness, and explain how to do one of them.
15. Give several examples of resistance in physical activity.

Ask the Author

Will girls build bigger muscles if they do muscle fitness exercises?

Get the answer and ask your own questions at the *Fitness for Life: Middle School* Web site.

Click Student Info ▶ Topic 7.11

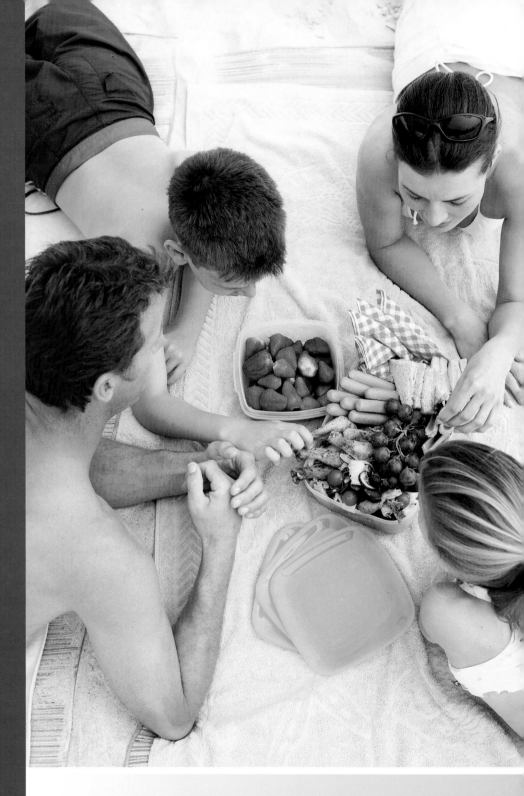

8

Body Composition, Physical Activity, and Nutrition

In this chapter...

Lesson 8.1

Body Composition

Lesson Vocabulary

body composition, body fatness, body mass index (BMI), calipers, eating disorder, essential fat, overweight, self-esteem

▶www.fitnessforlife.org/middleschool/
Click Student Info ▶ Topic 8.1

Body composition is one of the five parts of health-related physical fitness. Do you know what body composition is? Do you know what a healthy body composition is and how to tell if a person has it? When you finish this lesson, you'll know the answers to these questions. You'll also know some guidelines that can help you deal positively with peer pressure in physical activity.

What Is Body Composition?

Your body is made up of many different kinds of tissues including muscles, bones, fat, and organs. Each makes up a percentage of your total tissues, and together they describe the composition of your body. Many factors contribute to body composition including heredity, age, maturation, and healthy lifestyles such as physical activity and eating habits. You have no control over some of these factors, but you do have control over others. Physical activity and nutrition— two factors that you can control—are the focus of this chapter.

Body fat is one important component of body composition. Ideally, people shouldn't have too much or too little body fat. The goal is to be in the healthy fitness zone for **body fatness.** The best methods of assessing body fatness involve X-ray machines, electronic machines, and special water measurement tanks. But those pieces of equipment are expensive and can't be used quickly, so they aren't appropriate for general school classes. Instead, skinfold measurements are a good method for estimating your body fatness. They're not quite as

accurate, but they involve less equipment and are less expensive. To perform skinfold measurements, you need a pair of skinfold **calipers**—an instrument used to measure the thickness of fat folds beneath the skin. You also need a person who is trained in using the calipers, such as a trained partner or your physical education teacher.

Click Student Info ▶ Topic 8.2

Click Student Info ▶ Topic 8.2

FIT FACT

One of the most popular dolls in the United States is supposedly shaped like a young woman. But to have the doll's proportions, a real woman would have to be more than 7 feet (213 centimeters) tall and have a dangerously low level of body fat.

How Much Body Fat Should I Have?

Everyone needs to have some body fat. The minimum amount of fat necessary for good health is called **essential fat.** Fat is stored energy, and it can be used to provide fuel for physical activity. Having this source of energy would be especially important if you had to go without food for a long period of time. Body fat also acts as a shock absorber or as body padding, helping you keep from getting bruised when you get bumped. Fat also insulates your body and is especially useful in keeping you warm in cold temperatures.

Click Student Info ▶ Topic 8.3

Fat helps your body store and use vitamins. It also helps your body use hormones that are important to growth and other body functions. Having too little body fat can upset the normal functions of your body and lead to health problems.

Organs
Muscles
Fat
Bones

Your body is composed of many kinds of tissues.

Chapter 8 Body Composition, Physical Activity, and Nutrition **93**

Having too little body fat can also be a sign of an **eating disorder.** People with eating disorders typically eat too little and practice other poor nutrition habits; some exercise too much. Eating disorders can cause serious medical problems and often require the help of a professional. You can learn more about eating disorders, such as anorexia nervosa and bulimia, at the *Fitness for Life: Middle School* Web site.

Click Student Info ▶ Topic 8.4

Having too much body fat can also cause problems. People who have too much fat (also called being overfat) or have a high BMI (also called being overweight) have a greater risk of having diseases such as heart disease, cancer, and high blood pressure. Another disease called diabetes exists when the body's sugar levels are too high. People with this condition may need special medication and must pay particular attention to what they eat and how they exercise. The most common form of diabetes is much more frequent among people who have too much body fat. Medical costs are higher for people with too much body fat, and fatness can reduce a person's ability to work and play easily.

Boys typically have a lower percentage of body fat than girls do, especially in the later teen years. This is because boys have more of the male hormone that produces muscle growth. The hormone causes their bodies to have a higher percentage of muscle and a lower percentage of fat. As a result, boys and girls have different healthy fitness zone standards.

What Is the Body Mass Index?

You can also use your height and weight to calculate your **body mass index (BMI).** The BMI uses a formula to help you determine if you're overweight. The term **overweight** simply refers to having more weight than other people, which isn't the same as being high in body fat. It's possible to be high in weight without being too fat, because muscle weighs more than fat. People with a lot of muscle weigh more than people of the same size with less muscle. Nevertheless, the BMI gives you useful information related to health.

How Do I Determine My Body Fatness and BMI?

Read the "Skinfold Measurements" blue box on page 95 to learn how to measure skinfolds and how to determine your body fat levels using skinfold measurements. Tables 8.1 and 8.2 on page 98 will help you convert skinfold measurements to a percentage of body fat and help you to rate your body fat levels. Read the "Body Mass Index" blue box on page 96 to learn how to make height and weight measurements and how to determine your BMI using height and weight. Table 8.3 on page 98 will help you determine your BMI rating.

The BMI and skinfold measurement tests will help you determine if you are in the healthy fitness zone. Your test results will show if you're in a zone that helps you function effectively and avoid problems associated with having too much or too little body fat or body weight.

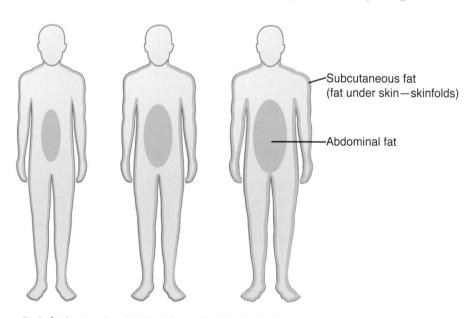

Subcutaneous fat
(fat under skin—skinfolds)

Abdominal fat

Body fat is stored under the skin and inside the body.

Many people feel that information about their body weight and body composition is personal. No matter what the reason, you have the right to treat your fitness testing results as private information. If people ask about your body weight, body composition, or other private information that you're not comfortable sharing, you can make a statement such as, "I don't feel comfortable sharing my personal information. Could you please respect my privacy?"

You should also help others keep their personal information private. For example, don't ask other people about their body weight or body composition. Also, if you work with a partner, keep his or her information private. In chapter 4, you learned some guidelines that you can use to build **self-esteem** (see pages 42–43). You may want to review those guidelines at this time.

You can take other steps to keep information confidential. One of the best ways is to share it only with people you trust, and only after asking them to keep the information private. Over time, you can build caring relationships with others, and this will reduce your need to worry about privacy. Sometimes, feeling comfortable in sharing information relieves the pressure of trying to keep things private.

Skinfold Measurements

You can use skinfold measurements to estimate body fat percentage. For teenagers, upper arm (triceps) and calf measurements provide a good estimate of body fat percentage. Work with a partner to take each other's measurements. When performing the skinfold measurements on your partner, use the instructions that follow.

Triceps skinfold: Pick up a skinfold on the middle of the back of the right arm, halfway between the elbow and the shoulder. The arm should hang loose and relaxed at the side.

Calf skinfold: The person being tested stands and places the right foot on a chair. Pick up a skinfold on the inside of the right calf halfway between the shin and the back of the calf, where the calf is largest.

1. Use your left thumb and index finger to pick up the skinfold. Do not pinch or squeeze the skinfold.

2. Hold the skinfold with your left hand while you pick up and use the caliper with the right hand to get a reading.

3. Place the caliper over the skinfold about one-half inch below your finger and thumb. Hold the caliper on the skinfold for 3 seconds, and then note the measurement. Read the caliper measurement to the nearest half millimeter (mm), if possible.

4. Make three measurements each for the triceps and the calf skinfolds. Use the middle of the three measures as the score. For example, an 8, 9, and 10 give a score of 9. If your three measurements differ by more than 2 mm, take a second or even third set of measurements.

Now you can determine your body fatness and fatness ratings. Add your triceps skinfold score and your calf skinfold score. Use table 8.1 to estimate your body fat percentage. For example, if you're a male and your skinfold sum is 27.5 mm, your body fat percentage is approximately 22 percent. Then look at table 8.2 to determine your rating for body fatness.

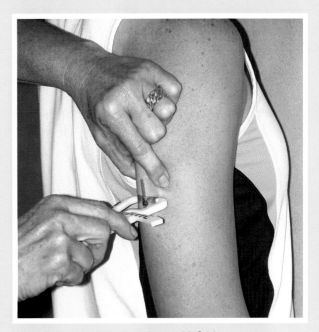

Use calipers to measure a triceps skinfold.

Adapted, by permission, from C. Corbin and R. Lindsey, 2005, *Fitness for life*, 5th ed. (Champaign, IL: Human Kinetics), 81.

Body Mass Index

As you measure your body mass index, use the worksheet supplied by your teacher to record your results and answer the questions about your BMI.

1. Measure your height in inches without shoes.

2. Measure your weight without shoes. If you're wearing street clothes (as opposed to lightweight gym clothing), subtract 2 pounds from your weight.

3. Use the body mass index chart to determine your BMI. You can also calculate your BMI using either of the following formulas:

   $$BMI = \text{weight in kilograms}/(\text{height in meters})^2$$

   $$BMI = \text{weight in pounds}/(\text{height in inches})^2 \times 703$$

4. Consult table 8.3 to find your BMI rating. Record the results on your worksheet.

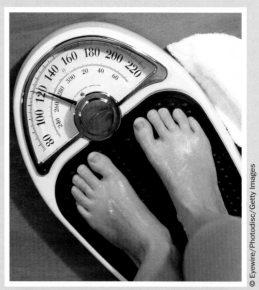

Height and weight measurements are used to determine BMI.

Height

Height \ Weight	70	75	80	85	90	95	100	105	110	115	120	125	130	135	140	145	150	155	160	165	170	175	180	185	190	195	200	205	210	215	220	225	230
4' 6"	17	18	19	20	22	23	24	25	27	28	29	30	31	32	34	35	36	37	39	40	41	42	43	45	46	47	48	49	51	52	53	54	56
4' 7"	16	17	19	20	21	22	23	24	26	27	28	29	30	31	32	34	35	36	37	38	39	40	41	43	45	46	47	48	49	50	51	52	54
4' 8"	16	17	18	19	20	21	22	24	25	26	27	28	29	30	31	32	34	35	36	37	38	39	40	42	43	44	45	46	47	48	49	50	52
4' 9"	15	16	17	18	19	21	22	23	24	25	26	27	28	29	30	31	32	34	35	36	37	38	39	40	42	42	43	44	45	47	48	49	50
4' 10"	15	16	17	18	19	20	21	22	23	24	25	26	27	28	29	30	31	32	34	35	36	37	38	39	40	41	42	43	44	45	46	47	48
4' 11"	14	15	16	17	18	20	20	21	22	23	24	25	26	27	28	29	30	31	32	33	34	35	36	37	38	39	40	41	42	43	45	46	46
5' 0"	14	15	16	17	18	19	19	21	22	22	23	24	25	26	27	28	29	30	31	32	33	34	35	36	37	38	39	40	41	42	43	44	45
5' 1"	13	14	15	16	17	18	19	20	21	22	23	24	25	26	26	27	28	29	30	31	32	33	34	35	36	37	38	39	40	41	42	43	43
5' 2"	13	14	15	16	17	17	18	19	20	21	22	23	24	25	26	27	27	28	29	30	31	32	33	34	35	36	37	37	38	39	40	41	42
5' 3"	12	13	14	15	16	17	18	19	19	21	21	22	23	24	25	26	27	27	28	29	30	31	32	33	34	35	35	36	37	38	39	40	41
5' 4"	12	13	14	15	15	16	17	18	19	20	20	21	22	23	24	25	26	27	27	28	29	30	31	32	33	33	34	35	36	37	38	39	39
5' 5"	12	12	13	14	15	16	17	18	18	20	20	21	22	22	23	24	25	26	27	27	28	29	30	31	32	32	33	34	35	36	37	37	38
5' 6"	11	12	13	14	15	15	16	17	18	19	19	20	21	22	23	24	25	25	26	27	27	28	29	30	31	31	32	33	34	35	36	36	37
5' 7"	11	12	13	13	14	15	16	17	17	19	19	20	20	21	22	23	23	24	25	26	27	27	28	29	30	31	31	32	33	34	34	35	36
5' 8"	11	11	12	13	14	14	15	16	17	18	19	20	20	21	21	22	23	24	24	25	26	27	27	28	29	30	30	31	32	33	33	34	35
5' 9"	10	11	12	13	13	14	15	16	16	18	18	18	19	20	21	21	22	23	24	24	25	26	27	27	28	29	30	30	31	32	32	33	34
5' 10"	10	11	11	12	13	14	14	15	16	17	17	18	19	19	20	21	22	22	23	24	24	25	26	27	27	28	29	29	30	31	32	32	33
5' 11"	10	11	11	12	13	13	14	15	15	17	17	17	18	19	20	20	21	22	22	23	24	24	25	26	26	27	28	28	29	30	31	31	32
6' 0"	9	10	11	12	12	13	14	14	15	16	16	17	18	18	19	20	20	21	22	22	23	24	24	25	26	26	27	28	28	29	30	31	31
6' 1"	9	10	11	11	12	13	13	14	15	15	16	16	17	18	18	19	20	20	21	22	22	23	24	24	25	26	26	27	28	28	29	30	30
6' 2"	9	10	10	11	12	12	13	13	14	15	15	16	17	17	18	19	19	20	21	21	22	22	23	24	24	25	26	26	27	28	28	29	30
6' 3"	9	9	10	11	11	12	13	13	14	15	15	16	16	17	18	18	19	19	20	21	21	22	22	24	24	24	25	26	26	27	27	28	29
6' 4"	8	9	10	10	11	12	12	13	13	14	15	15	16	16	17	18	18	19	20	20	21	21	22	23	23	24	24	25	26	26	27	27	28

Weight

Adapted, by permission, from C. Corbin and R. Lindsey, 2005, *Fitness for Life*, 5th ed. (Champaign, IL: Human Kinetics), 226-227.

Moving Together: Peer Pressure

Do you ever feel pressured to do things that you don't feel comfortable doing? Is it hard sometimes to do activities that you like when others call them dumb? It can be hard to make friends with someone if other people think that person is weird.

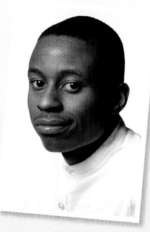

Mel was on the community soccer team. He enjoyed being on the team and liked to play soccer. Mel knew that the physical activity that he got when he played soccer was good for him, and he knew that his parents expected him to be at practice when he told them he would. Sometimes Mel's friends who didn't play on the soccer team tried to talk him out of going to practice. His friends didn't eat lunch and saved their lunch money to play games at a video arcade after school. They spent a lot of time hanging out without really doing much. They put a lot of pressure on Mel to skip practice and be with them. One of the teens in the group told Mel that he needed to decide whether he wanted to be friends with him or with the kids on the soccer team. Mel had a problem because he wanted to play on the soccer team but he also wanted to be with his friends.

Discussion Questions

1. What can Mel do to solve his problem?
2. Are there people Mel can talk to who can help him?
3. Are there ways that Mel can be on the soccer team and have friends who aren't on the team?
4. Should Mel give in to the pressure of his peers? How can he deal with this pressure?

Guidelines for Making Choices With Friends

▶ *Identify the problem and identify possible solutions.* Before making a decision and taking a course of action, clarify the exact nature of the problem. Then make a list of possible solutions. Talking to a parent or teacher may help you identify problems and possible solutions associated with making choices with friends.

▶ *Determine the good things about different choices.* If you have several choices and they seem to conflict, make a list of the good things that will happen if you make each choice. This will help you see the benefits of making one choice or another.

▶ *Determine the negative things about different choices.* Just as there are good things that will happen if you make different choices, there may be some negative things as well. Listing the negatives can help you make a good choice.

▶ *Discuss possible solutions with people you trust.* Discussing your choices with a parent, a teacher, or another older person can help you see good things and bad things about each choice that you might not have seen on your own.

▶ *Talk to your friends about your goals and theirs.* When making choices that involve friends, it's important to know what their goals are. You can share your goals (as well as the good and bad things about different choices) to see if your goals are similar to your friends' goals.

▶ *Choose friends whose goals are similar to yours.* If you choose friends who have similar positive goals, they can help support your choices (and you can support theirs).

▶ *Use "I statements" to express yourself.* It helps to use "I statements" that express your feelings and let others know you care about their feelings. For example, Mel might say, "I'm mixed up because I really enjoy hanging with you guys, but soccer is really important to me." Or he could say, "I hear you saying you want me to hang with you guys all the time and give up soccer, but I really want to do both. Maybe I can do stuff with you on Saturdays, and I can hit soccer practice during the week."

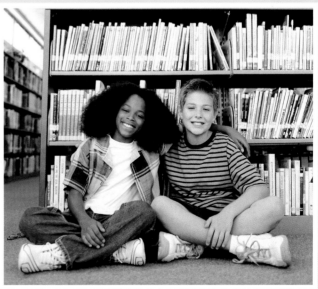

Good friends have similar positive goals and support each other.

© Image Source

Click Student Info ▶ Topic 8.5

Table 8.1

Converting Skinfold Measurements to Percentage of Body Fat

MALES		FEMALES	
Sum	%	Sum	%
12	10	19.5	17
13.5	11	21	18
15	12	23	19
16.5	13	24.5	20
18	14	26	21
19	16	27.5	22
20.5	17	29.5	23
22	18	31	24
23	19	32.5	25
24.5	19	34.5	26
26	20	36	27
27	21	37.5	28
28.5	22	39.5	29
30	23	41	30
31	24	42.5	31
32.5	25	44	32

Data generated from Fitnessgram software.

Take It Home

Give Me a Commercial Break

"Get fit in 5 minutes a day!" "Lose 10 pounds in a week!" We're constantly bombarded with commercials that make false claims. Movie stars try to get you to buy products that they might not even use. Some of the people who appear in commercials might not look the same way in real life. Computers are often used to change the way people look and to make them appear thinner than they really are. Unrealistic pictures of men with huge muscles and women who are exceptionally thin are common. You might not realize it, but these commercials can affect how we feel about ourselves.

Have you ever really checked out the commercials you see on TV or hear on the radio? How about the advertisements you see in magazines or on billboards? What messages are they trying to send? Analyzing commercials and advertisements can help you become an informed consumer about physical activity and nutrition.

Becoming an informed consumer takes practice. Use the worksheet supplied by your teacher to analyze three commercials that you see during your favorite TV program. What strategies do the commercials use to sell their products? What other messages do they send?

Click Student Info ▶ Topic 8.6

Table 8.2

Body Fat Ratings

Age	Needs improvement	Healthy fitness zone	Very lean*
MALES			
All ages	More than 25%	25–10%	9.9% or less
FEMALES			
All ages	More than 32%	32–17%	16.9% or less

*Scores in the very lean category may not be best for good health.

Data generated from Fitnessgram software.

Table 8.3

Body Mass Index (BMI) Ratings

Age	Needs improvement	Healthy fitness zone	Very lean*
MALES			
10	21.1 or more	21–15.3	15.2 or less
11	21.1 or more	21–15.8	15.7 or less
12	22.1 or more	22–16	15.9 or less
13	23.1 or more	23–16.6	16.5 or less
14	24.6 or more	24.5–17.5	17.4 or less
15+	25.1 or more	25–18.1	18.0 or less
FEMALES			
10	23.6 or more	23.5–16.6	16.5 or less
11	24.1 or more	24–16.9	16.8 or less
12	24.6 or more	24.5–16.9	16.8 or less
13	24.6 or more	24.5–17.5	17.4 or less
14	25.1 or more	25–17.5	17.4 or less
15+	25.1 or more	25–17.5	17.4 or less

*Scores in the very lean category may not be best for good health.

Data generated from Fitnessgram software.

Lesson Review

▶ What is body composition?

▶ How do you know whether a person has a healthy body composition?

▶ What is BMI?

▶ Describe some guidelines for making choices with friends.

Energy Balance: Physical Activity and Nutrition

Lesson Vocabulary

basal metabolism, calories, carbohydrates, discretionary foods, efficiency, energy balance, energy expenditure, energy intake, fats, minerals, MyPyramid, nutrients, protein, vitamins

Click Student Info ▶ Topic 8.7

Energy balance is important to having a healthy body composition. Do you know what energy balance means? Do you know how to eat well for maintaining energy balance and for good health? How does physical activity affect energy balance? When you finish this lesson, you'll know the answers to these questions. You'll also know the importance of efficiency to your performance in physical activity.

What Is Energy Balance?

Energy balance means consuming only as much energy through food as your body uses each day. One way to measure energy is to count the **calories** contained in the food you eat. These calories are what your body burns when you exercise. The calorie content of the food you eat is called **energy intake**, and the calories that your body burns is referred to as **energy expenditure.**

The typical teenage girl burns about 2,200 calories each day, and the typical teenage boy burns about 2,800 calories a day. This amount varies based on age,

body size, heredity, and daily activity level. To have energy balance, a person must expend the same number of calories that she or he consumes each day. People who take in more calories than they expend will gain weight, and people who take in fewer calories than they expend will lose weight. Inactive teens need to consume fewer calories to maintain energy balance. Active teens involved in dance, sports, and other activities need to consume more calories each day than less active teens.

What Should I Eat?

MyPyramid is a food guide developed by the United States Department of Agriculture to help you consume the right amounts of food and the right kinds of food. As you already learned, the calories you take in should balance the calories you expend. But there are other important reasons for choosing foods. Food provides not only energy but also other important **nutrients** such as carbohydrates, protein, and fat—the three major sources of calories. Food also provides **vitamins** and **minerals** that are necessary to keep you healthy and to help your body function efficiently.

Click Student Info ▶ Topic 8.8

MyPyramid has colored bands that represent various types of food. The wider the color band in MyPyramid, the more servings of that type of food you should eat. The orange band represents grains, the green band represents vegetables, and the red band represents fruits. Grains, vegetables, and fruits are the primary sources of **carbohydrates** and should

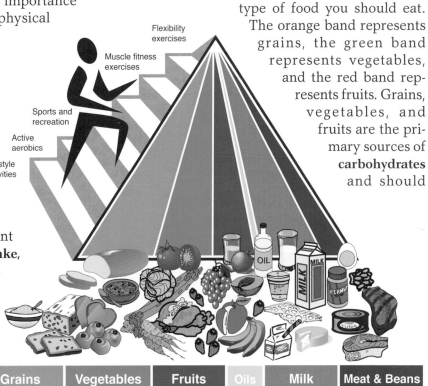

Flexibility exercises
Muscle fitness exercises
Sports and recreation
Active aerobics
Lifestyle activities

| Grains | Vegetables | Fruits | Oils | Milk | Meat & Beans |

MyPyramid is a guide to healthy eating and healthy exercise.

Reprinted, by permission, from C. Corbin and R. Lindsey, 2007, *Fitness for Life*, updated 5th ed. (Champaign, IL: Human Kinetics), 247.

be a big part of your diet. Carbohydrates are forms of sugar and fiber. There are two types of carbohydrates, simple and complex. Simple carbohydrates (sugars such as those in candy and soft drinks) should be limited in your diet, but complex carbohydrates provide vitamins and energy for daily activities. Complex carbohydrates (such as those in whole grains and many fruits and vegetables) also provide fiber that aids in digestion. Each day, teens should consume several servings of whole grains, as well as three or more servings of fruit and four or more servings of vegetables.

The blue band in MyPyramid represents milk products, and the purple band represents meat and beans. These foods are high in **protein.** Your body needs protein from these foods to build muscle and other body tissues. Milk products are also high in calcium, a mineral necessary to build strong bones. However, milk, meat, and beans are sometimes high in fat, so it's best to choose low-fat or nonfat milk products and lean cuts of meat. You need two or three servings from each of these two groups.

As noted earlier, **fats** are present in many foods. Fats that are solid at room temperature and that are typically made from animal products are called saturated fats. These products, such as butter, should be used sparingly. Fats that are not solid at room temperature, such as many oils, are more healthful,

Calories in foods that are high in simple sugar (such as soda and candy) are called "empty calories" because they do little for health and wellness.

especially fish oil, canola oil, and olive oil. Oils that are converted to solid form, such as margarine, are called trans fats. Like saturated fats, they should be limited in your diet.

One type of food isn't represented in MyPyramid because foods in this group aren't necessary for good nutrition. These **discretionary foods** include mustard, ketchup, dressings, and sauces. You can use some of these foods to make healthy food taste better, but like oils, they're often high in calories, so use them in moderation.

The word "dieting" often refers to limiting the number of calories consumed, usually to lose excess body fat (which is often referred to as "losing weight"). However, teens shouldn't restrict their calorie intake too much. If you take in too few calories, you won't get enough of the basic nutrients that are needed for good health and for the cells of your body to work properly. As noted earlier in the chapter, eating too little can cause health problems and could lead to an eating disorder. Teens who are considering cutting calories should prepare a good eating plan to be sure that they still get the nutrients they need. Advice from parents and experts is recommended to help teens have a healthy diet and avoid health problems.

Click Student Info ▶ Topic 8.9

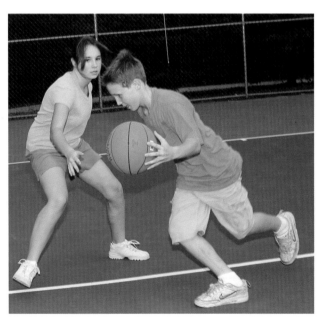
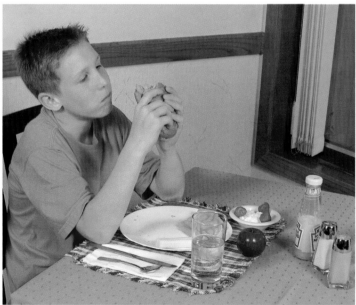

After expending energy in physical activity, eating nutritious food helps restore your energy balance.

Biomechanical Principles: Efficiency

Part of learning to move skillfully is learning to move without wasted or unnecessary energy.

Efficiency is the ability to perform in the best possible way with little wasted energy. Calories from food give us the energy to do physical activity. We use the energy to contract the muscles. The muscle contractions move the body levers and cause movement. For efficiency, we try to conserve energy or use the least energy possible to accomplish the task we are performing.

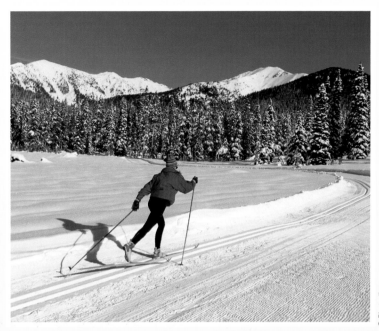

Efficiency helps a skier conserve energy in a long race.

© Photodisc

to be quite as efficient as when you're trying to win a race. Also, you can add resistance to expend more calories. For example, when you carry a backpack, you expend more energy than when you walk without one. Carrying a backpack in a race would cause you to expend extra energy but would slow you down and make you less likely to win the race.

Being efficient is important when doing a job because if you don't use a lot of energy, you can do the job for a long time without getting tired. In physical activities such as skiing in a long race, efficiency is also important. A cross-country skier who skis efficiently conserves energy and has a better chance of winning a race than a skier who is inefficient. The biomechanical principles you studied earlier in this book help you to be efficient in movement. For example, if you apply force in the right direction when walking and running, you'll be more efficient than if you apply force in other directions. If you use your body's levers properly, you move more efficiently. No matter what activity you choose, you can learn to be more efficient by applying biomechanical principles. Practice is also important to improve efficiency, because it helps you eliminate wasted movements.

Sometimes, you might want to be inefficient and use more energy rather than less energy. For example, playing in a pool and swimming in an inefficient manner will expend more calories than swimming efficiently. This inefficient activity expends many calories and helps balance the energy you consume in food.

Food provides the energy you need to be active, but if you eat too much food, the extra energy (calories) will be stored in your body as fat. When you do physical activity, you use this extra energy (extra calories). So to maintain a healthy body weight, you may not want

Applying the Principle

Describe what you can do to improve efficiency (conserve energy) when performing the following activities. Then describe which activities would be best for helping you maintain a healthy body weight by expending calories.

▶ Swimming
▶ Running
▶ Walking
▶ Resistance exercises
▶ Soccer
▶ Digging in a garden
▶ Watching TV

Principles in Practice

Use table 8.4 (page 102) to determine how much energy you expend in typical activities. Practice techniques that allow you to become more efficient while doing those activities. In addition, try to be aware of calories that you take in. For example, one regular 12-ounce (355-milliliter) soft drink contains approximately 150 calories of energy. Each time you drink a can of soda, perform several activities from table 8.4 to expend the energy you just consumed.

Click Student Info ▶ **Topic 8.10**

Table 8.4

Energy (Calories per Hour) Expended in Various Activities*

Light activity	Calories	Moderate activity	Calories	Vigorous activity	Calories
Lying down	78	Bowling	176	Biking (10 mph or 16 km/h)	311
Sitting	85	Sweeping	198	Playing basketball	360
Reading	90	Horseback riding	204	Aerobic dance	438
Playing cards	105	Biking (7 mph or 11.2 km/h)	210	Soccer	459
Typing	110	Golf	212	Racquetball	510
Playing computer games	120	Raking leaves	230	Swimming fast	530
Washing dishes	135	Walking (3.5 mph or 5.6 km/h)	240	Running (10 mph or 16 km/h)	595

*Calories are for a 120-pound (54-kilogram) person. Amounts are less for lighter people and more for heavier people.

How Active Should I Be to Balance Energy?

Your body expends calories when you're not active, even if you're just sitting, lying, or sleeping. This is because your heart and other body organs require energy to do their work. The amount of energy necessary just to keep your body going is called your **basal metabolism.**

Metabolism refers to the process of converting food to energy. *Basal* means "basic." As shown in table 8.4, you also use energy in light activities such as brushing your teeth, reading a book, sitting and standing, and participating in sports and games.

Moderate activities such as those in level 1 of the Physical Activity Pyramid expend more calories than light activities. Vigorous activities at levels 2 and 3 of the Physical Activity Pyramid expend even more calories. Labels from the Physical Activity Pyramid are included by the stairway in MyPyramid to show you that both activity and good nutrition are important to energy balance.

As shown in table 8.4, very active people expend a lot of calories. For example, a volleyball player burns calories not only during a game, but also during practices and training while preparing for a game. Progressive resistance exercises that are done to build muscle expend calories, but they also contribute to the calories that a person expends at rest. This is because resistance exercises build muscles, and muscles burn more calories than other tissues such as fat, even when the body is resting.

Because vigorous exercise expends more calories in a short period of time, teens sometimes think this is the best type of activity for weight control. To be sure, vigorous activity can be an important part of an overall activity plan, but moderate activity can be a great way to expend calories because it can be done for long periods of time without stopping. Some people—especially those who don't play sports—find it easier to do moderate activity rather than vigorous activity on a regular basis. You can try out some tools that can help you maintain your energy balance at the *Fitness for Life: Middle School* Web site.

Click Student Info ▶ Topic 8.11

Just as you should have a good plan if you want to reduce your calorie intake, you should also have a good plan if you want to do additional activity to expend more energy. You'll learn more about how to develop a plan in the next chapter.

Lesson Review

- ▶ What is energy balance?
- ▶ How should you eat to be healthy and maintain energy balance?
- ▶ How is efficiency important to performance in physical activity?
- ▶ How is physical activity important to energy balance?

8

Chapter Review

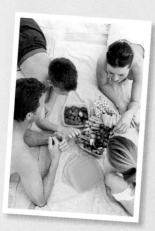

Number your paper from 1 to 5. Read each question. After the number for the question, write a word or a phrase that best answers the question. The page number where you can find the answer is listed after the question.

1. What two words are used to describe the types of tissues that make up the body? (page 93)

2. What word describes a condition that exists when your body weight is higher than it should be for good health? (page 94)

3. What three letters are used as an abbreviation for one of the measurements of body composition contained in Fitnessgram? (page 94)

4. What term describes ketchup, mustard, and other foods not represented in the main categories of MyPyramid? (page 100)

5. What term describes the amount of energy used by the body when it's inactive? (page 102)

Number your paper from 6 to 10. Next to each number, write the letter of the best answer.

6. bulimia
7. calorie
8. calipers
9. carbohydrate
10. protein

a. a unit of energy contained in food
b. a tool used to measure skinfold thickness
c. a nutrient found in fruits and vegetables
d. a type of eating disorder
e. a nutrient found in meat and beans

Number your paper from 11 to 15. Follow the directions to answer each question or statement.

11. Give reasons why it's important to have some body fat.

12. Give examples of guidelines for dealing with peer pressure in positive ways.

13. Draw a picture of MyPyramid, and give examples of the foods represented in the pyramid.

14. Explain what is meant by energy balance and why it's important to body composition.

15. Discuss efficiency and give examples of how it's important in physical activity and daily life.

Ask the Authors

Is it possible to be physically fit and still be fat?
 Get the answer and ask your own questions at the *Fitness for Life: Middle School* Web site.

Click Student Info ▶ Topic 8.12

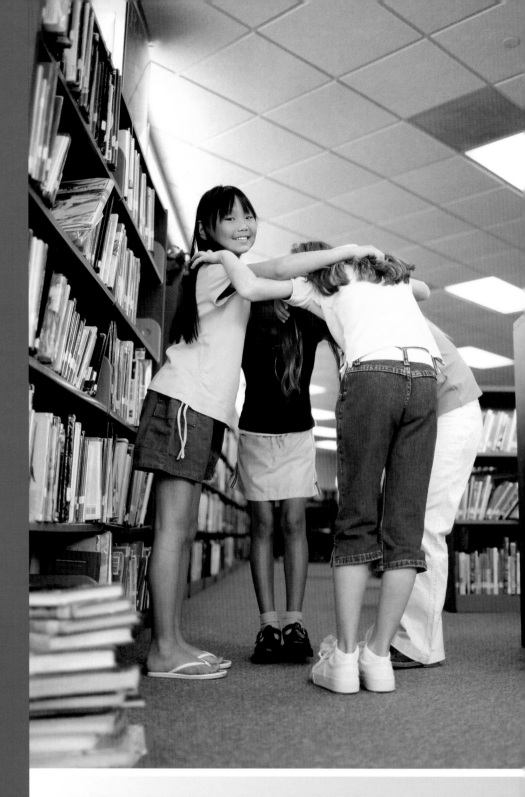

9

Planning for Physical Activity

Self-Assessing Fitness and Physical Activity Needs

Lesson Vocabulary

fitness summary, physical activity summary

▶ **www.fitnessforlife.org/middleschool/**
Click Student Info ▶ Topic 9.1

Young kids often have little choice about what they do in life. To be sure, there are some things that teens can't control, but in general, teens make more and more of their own decisions as they grow older. You get to choose whether you'll take care of your body and make healthy decisions or not.

Building a fitness summary and a physical activity summary can help you create a physical activity plan that can lead to a long, enjoyable, healthy life. Do you know how fit and active you are? Do you have the information you need to assess your fitness and activity levels and to build a fitness summary and a physical activity summary? When you finish this lesson, you'll know the answers to these questions. You'll also know some guidelines for becoming fit and active.

How Fit Am I?

Some people see fitness tests as something that they have to do because the teacher says so, but they feel the tests aren't really important. However, knowing how fit you are helps you analyze your own needs and take positive control of your own health. A good way to keep track of your fitness is to build a **fitness summary.** The summary is a written record of your fitness test scores and ratings. It helps you determine your strength and weaknesses. Table 9.1 shows a sample fitness summary for Keisha, who did all of the Fitnessgram self-assessments during her class. Over the summer Keisha was very active, so at the end of the summer she did a reassessment to see if she had improved her fitness. You can see the results of Keisha's reassessment in table 9.1, too.

Click Student Info ▶ Topic 9.2

You'll have the opportunity to use a worksheet to build your own fitness summary using the results of the self-assessments you have already performed. You might be able to enter your results in the computer to prepare a Fitnessgram report if you choose (see page 10). When you finish your fitness summary or a Fitnessgram report, you'll know whether you're physically fit. If you need to improve your fitness in any areas, you can decide how to accomplish that goal. Analyzing your own fitness can be an empowering activity.

As you can tell from looking at Keisha's fitness summary, it's possible to be fit in one area but not so fit in another. The first time Keisha took the Fitnessgram self-assessments, she needed improvement in three areas, but she was in the healthy fitness zone in all other areas. When she did the follow-up assessment after a summer of regular physical activity, she was in the healthy fitness zones in all areas of fitness.

Table 9.1

Keisha's Fitness Summary

TYPE OF TEST	SELF-ASSESSMENT		REASSESSMENT	
	Score	**Rating**	**Score**	**Rating**
PACER	28 laps	Healthy fitness zone	41 laps	Healthy fitness zone
Sit-and-reach				
Right	10 inches (25.4 centimeters)	Healthy fitness zone	12 inches (30.5 centimeters)	Healthy fitness zone
Left	8 inches (20.3 centimeters)	Needs improvement	10 inches (25.4 centimeters)	Healthy fitness zone
Trunk lift	12 inches (30.5 centimeters)	Healthy fitness zone	12 inches (30.5 centimeters)	Healthy fitness zone
Curl-up	15	Needs improvement	20	Healthy fitness zone
Push-up	6	Needs improvement	8	Healthy fitness zone
BMI	22.5	Healthy fitness zone	21.5	Healthy fitness zone
Percent fat	25	Healthy fitness zone	23	Healthy fitness zone

How Active Am I?

A **physical activity summary** lets you know how active you are. The summary includes all of the types of physical activity from the Physical Activity Pyramid. Table 9.2 shows a physical activity summary for Keisha. She answered five questions related to the five types of physical activity included in the Physical Activity Pyramid. Then she did a follow-up assessment at the end of the summer.

You'll have the opportunity to answer the same questions Keisha answered. Your answers will provide a summary of your normal activity level each week. Use the worksheet provided by your teacher to do your own physical activity summary. With the help of your teacher, you may also want to create an Activitygram report that summarizes the type and amount of activity you perform. Are you physically active enough for good health? Your activity summary will help you answer that question. You may be active in one area but not so active in another.

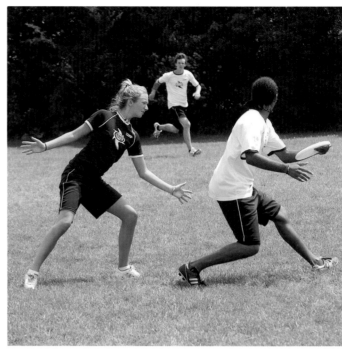

Make sure that your plan includes activities that you really enjoy.

How Active Are Teens?

Teens from all over the United States were asked to do a physical activity assessment, much like the one that Keisha did. They answered the questions based on their activity in the previous seven days.

Table 9.2

Keisha's Physical Activity Summary*

ACTIVITY QUESTION	SELF-ASSESSMENT		REASSESSMENT	
	Yes	No	Yes	No
Do you do 30 or more minutes of **lifestyle physical activity** at least five days a week? (See chapter 3.)	✓		✓	
Do you do **active aerobic activities** that elevate your heart rate into the target zone for 20 minutes a day at least three days a week? (See chapter 4.)	✓		✓	
Do you do **active sports and recreation activities** that elevate your heart rate into the target zone for 20 minutes a day at least three days a week? (See chapter 5.)		✓	✓	
Do you do **flexibility exercises** at least three days a week? (See chapter 6.)		✓	✓	
Do you do **muscle fitness exercises** at least two days a week? (See chapter 7.)		✓	✓	

*Answer the questions based on the last seven days. If your activity over the last seven days is not typical of your normal activity, answer the questions based on a normal week.

- Teens were asked if they did 30 or more minutes of lifestyle physical activity at least five days a week. Only 27% of males said yes, and only 22% of females answered yes.
- Teens were asked if they did active aerobic activities at least three days a week. To qualify as an active aerobic activity, the activity had to

FIT FACT

Losing weight is a common New Year's resolution—adults in the United States buy more gym memberships in January than during any other month. Unfortunately, less than half are still exercising after six months, and less than 10 percent are still exercising after a year.

elevate their heart rate into the target zone for 20 minutes a day. However, the question didn't specify the type of vigorous activity, so teens could include active aerobics, active sports, and active recreation activities in their response. This time, 70% of males answered yes, and 55% of females answered yes.

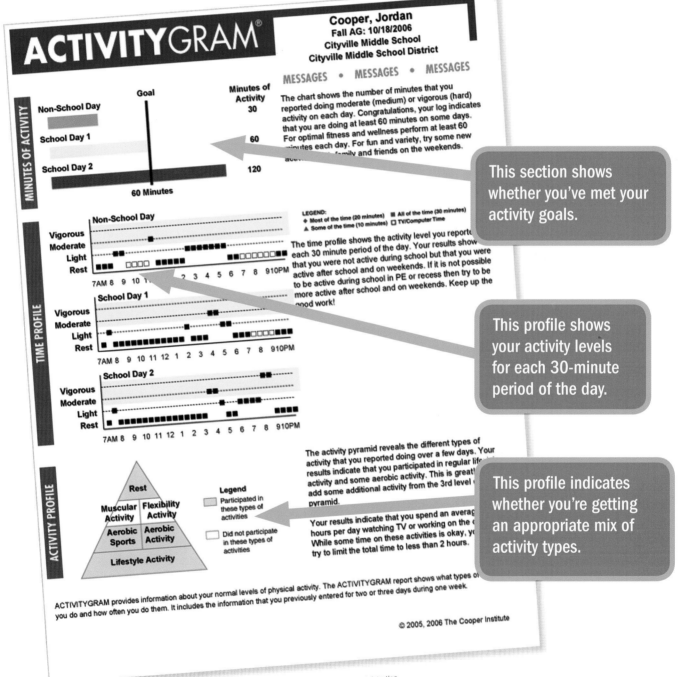

This section shows whether you've met your activity goals.

This profile shows your activity levels for each 30-minute period of the day.

This profile indicates whether you're getting an appropriate mix of activity types.

Adapted, by permission, from The Cooper Institute, 2005, *Fitnessgram/Activitygram test administration manual*, updated 4th ed. (Champaign, IL: Human Kinetics).

You can do an Activitygram to summarize your level of physical activity.

Moving Together: Getting Active and Fit

What parts of your physical fitness do you want to improve? Why? What kinds of activities can you see yourself participating in to improve your fitness? When you think about these activities, do you see yourself participating for competition or fun? Will you participate alone, with friends, with family, on a team, or in some combination of these? Will you participate outdoors, indoors, or both?

Earlier in this lesson you learned about Keisha. Keisha had done all of the Fitnessgram tests and prepared a fitness summary. She also prepared a physical activity summary. After doing the fitness tests for the first time, Keisha decided that she wanted to be more active and to try to improve her fitness so that she could score in the healthy fitness zone in all areas of fitness. She prepared a plan and carried it out over the summer. When she reassessed her fitness at the end of the summer, she found that she had met her goal. Keisha used her fitness information to make important decisions that helped her to meet her goals.

LaBrea also did a fitness summary after taking all of the Fitnessgram self-assessments. He found that he needed improvement in many areas of fitness. LaBrea needed improvement in cardiovascular fitness and muscle fitness (as shown in his results on the push-up test). His BMI score indicated that he needed improvement as well. He scored in the healthy fitness zone for curl-ups, the sit-and-reach, and the trunk lift.

As you might imagine, LaBrea also needed to become more active. He was only able to say yes to one of the questions in table 9.2. However, he already did stretching exercises on most days of the week. From what he had learned in previous lessons, he knew that he needed to be more active. But LaBrea knew that his parents weren't as fit as they should be, and he thought that maybe there was nothing he could do about his own fitness.

Discussion Questions

1. LaBrea thinks that he might not be able to change his fitness. Do you think that this is true?

2. LaBrea needs to make important decisions about his lack of fitness and physical activity. What are some of the first steps he should take?

3. Why do you think Keisha was successful in becoming more active and carrying out her plan?

4. What other advice could you give to LaBrea to get him going? What other advice could you give to Keisha to keep her going?

Guidelines for Getting Active and Fit

▶ *Determine your needs.* Before you can make good decisions, you need good information. Preparing a fitness summary and a physical activity summary will give you information about your fitness and activity levels and what you need to do to improve them. Compare your results with the recommendations for your age group. See if you're in the healthy fitness zone for all the fitness components.

▶ *Set SMART goals.* Once you know your fitness and activity needs, you can set personal goals to meet those needs. Setting SMART goals can help. You will learn about SMART goals in the next lesson.

▶ *Develop a sound plan.* Follow the steps on page 111 to prepare an activity plan that is based on your SMART goals. Developing a plan helps you take action. A good plan includes the activities you'll do and a schedule for when you'll do them.

▶ *Keep track of your progress.* Once you've developed a plan, keep records. For example, keeping a log or diary can help you stick with your plan. You can also reassess your level of fitness from time to time. Experts suggest giving yourself time to improve before doing a reassessment. Making assessments too often can be discouraging because it takes several weeks for a good activity plan to show results.

▶ *Seek support from others.* The encouragement and support of other people makes it easier to stick to a plan. Asking family members and friends for support and encouragement is a good idea. Even better is finding family and friends to be active with you. People stick to their activity plans much better when they've made a commitment to someone else.

▶ *Don't expect too much too soon. Keep giving effort.* Sometimes people expect instant improvement. As you learned earlier, it takes time to make changes in most things. Effort is the key! If you stick with your plan and keep trying, over the long term you'll see improvement.

Click Student Info ▶ Topic 9.3

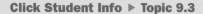

- The assessment didn't ask questions about flexibility exercises, so there is no data about the percentage of activity in that area.
- Teens were asked if they did muscle fitness exercises at least two days a week. In response, 60% of males and 43% of females answered yes.

As you can see, more boys than girls get the recommended amount of exercise. More teens meet the national standard for vigorous activity than other types of activity listed. Experts are concerned about the fact that 33 percent of teens don't get enough activity to build good health and fitness, and 12 percent get no regular activity at all.

Take It Home

Moving Forward

Even though you have already learned a lot, your journey to a healthy and active lifestyle is just beginning. Active participation in this class has given you many of the skills you need to become physically active on your own. For example, you can self-assess your physical fitness levels, find opportunities for physical activity in your neighborhood, set goals for activity, and reflect on your feelings about physical activity. You have also learned about and practiced valuable skills that will help you to be active and to encourage others to lead healthy lifestyles. For example, you have practiced communication skills, teamwork skills, and strategies to help others make healthy changes in behavior.

Use the worksheet supplied by your teacher to plan for physical activity with a member of your support team. Maybe the plan will help you become more active, or maybe it will help the other person become more active. Either way, you'll continue your journey to active living, good health, and happiness with your family and friends.

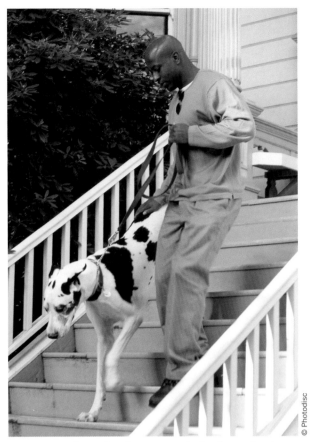

Adults meet the national recommendation for moderate activity more often than teens.

Lesson Review

- ▶ How do you assess your fitness and build a fitness summary?
- ▶ How do you assess your activity level and build a physical activity summary?
- ▶ Describe some guidelines for becoming active and fit and staying active and fit.

Creating a Physical Activity Plan

Your fitness and activity summaries can help you determine your fitness and activity needs and establish your personal fitness goals. Do you know what your fitness and activity needs are? Do you know how to establish goals? Do you know how to develop a physical activity plan? When you finish this lesson, you'll know the answers to these questions. You'll also understand how integrating biomechanical principles is important to your performance in physical activity.

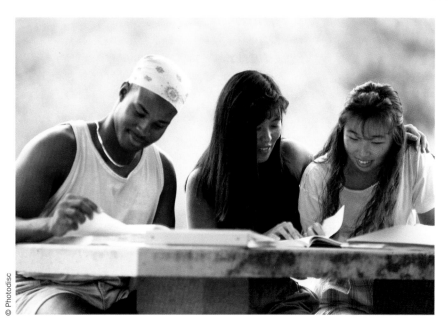

The first step in creating a physical activity plan is identifying your fitness and activity needs.

© Photodisc

What Are My Fitness and Activity Needs?

Earlier you learned how Keisha prepared a fitness summary and a physical activity summary to help identify her areas of need. Keisha's needs based on her summaries are shown in table 9.3 and table 9.4. You can use similar tables to help you identify areas of fitness that need improvement and determine if you need more activity of a certain type. Keisha's initial fitness summary showed that she needed improvement in flexibility and muscle fitness. It's not surprising that Keisha didn't answer "yes" for getting enough flexibility and muscle fitness exercise since her fitness scores needed improvement in these areas. Keisha also didn't do as much active sports and recreation as experts recommend.

What Are My Fitness and Activity Goals?

Keisha made a list of her short-term physical activity goals. **Short-term goals** can be reached in a few days or weeks. Experts suggest focusing on short-term physical activity goals when you first start a program. For example, you could set a short-term goal of doing lifestyle activity or muscle fitness exercises three days a week. To reach this short-term goal, you need to do the exercises on a regular basis for a set amount of time, such as three weeks.

Once you have met this short-term goal, you can set another. Reaching a series of short-term goals can help you reach your long-term fitness goals. Effort is the key to reaching short-term goals. If you make the effort to do the exercises, you'll meet your goal.

Long-term goals take many weeks, and often several months, to reach. Fitness goals aren't suggested as short-term goals, but they can be used as long-term goals. This is because building fitness takes time. In most cases, it takes at least six weeks of regular activity before you'll see changes in your fitness scores. If you meet a series of short-term physical activity goals as described in the previous paragraph, and if they're appropriate goals, you'll ultimately reach your long-term fitness goals.

If you set a fitness goal—for example, increasing the number of push-ups you can do—as a short-term goal, you may become discouraged because you won't be able to meet the goal in a short period of time. On the other hand, anyone can give the effort necessary to achieve physical activity goals, and regular physical activity is required for building fitness, so activity goals are especially good for the short term.

SMART goals are the best goals. *SMART* is a term that helps you remember five important characteristics of fitness and activity goals.

- S stands for specific.
- M stands for measurable.
- A stands for attainable.
- R stands for reasonable.
- T stands for timely.

After Keisha determined her fitness and activity needs (tables 9.3 and 9.4), she was ready to set some SMART short-term activity goals (table 9.5). Using a worksheet, she set a goal of performing several different activities from the Physical Activity Pyramid for a period of four weeks. To make the goals specific, she listed the activities that she planned to do on her worksheet. To make sure that the goals were measurable, she indicated the amount of time she wanted to do them and the numbers of days she planned to do the activities each week. She selected only as many activities as she thought she could reasonably do on a regular basis. She wanted to be sure that her goals were attainable. She knew her goals were timely because

the activities she chose were good for meeting her fitness and activity needs. Because Keisha was just beginning her program, she focused on short-term physical activity goals.

Click Student Info ▶ Topic 9.5

What Is a Physical Activity Plan?

A good physical activity plan is a written list of specific activities that you will perform, along with a schedule of when you'll do them. By adding the time of day to her list of activity goals, Keisha came up with a four-week activity plan (see table 9.6).

Table 9.3

Keisha's Fitness Needs

Type of fitness	Needs improvement
Cardiovascular fitness	
Flexibility	✓
Muscle fitness	✓
Body composition	

Table 9.4

Keisha's Physical Activity Needs

Type of activity	Needs improvement
Lifestyle activity	
Active aerobics	
Active sports and recreation	✓
Flexibility exercise	✓
Muscle fitness exercise	✓

Table 9.5

Keisha's Short-Term Activity Goals

Type of activity	Short-term activity goals
Lifestyle activity	Begin doing 30 minutes per day, six days a week.
Active aerobics and active sports and recreation	Maintain current activity, doing either active aerobics or active sports and recreation three days a week for 20 minutes in the target heart rate zone.
Flexibility exercise	Begin doing five basic stretching exercises five days a week.
Muscle fitness exercise	Begin doing five basic muscle fitness exercises three days a week.

Table 9.6

Keisha's Short-Term Activity Goals and Personal Activity Plan

Type of activity	Name of activity	Minutes per day	Days per week	Start/end time
Lifestyle activity	Walking	15	(M) T (W) Th (F) (S) (Su)	7:30 to 7:45 a.m.
	Walking	15	(M) T (W) Th (F) (S) (Su)	Noon to 12:15 p.m.
Active aerobics	Aerobic dance	30	M (T) W (Th) F S Su	4:00 to 4:30 p.m.
Active sports or recreation	Tennis	60	M T W Th F S (Su)	6:00 to 7:00 p.m.

Type of activity	Name of exercise	Reps (Number/length)	Days per week	Time of day
Flexibility exercise	Sit and reach	3 for 30 seconds	M (T) W (Th) F S (Su)	After warming up for tennis and aerobic dance
	Calf stretch	3 for 30 seconds		
	Chest stretch	3 for 30 seconds		
	Hip stretch	3 for 30 seconds		
	Knee to chest stretch	3 for 30 seconds		

Type of activity	Name of exercise	Number of sets and reps	Days per week	Time of day
Muscle fitness exercise	Curl-ups	3 and 10	(M) T (W) Th (F) S Su	Before bed
	Push-ups	3 and 10		
	Arm circles	3 and 10		
	Two-leg press*	3 and 10		
	Leg curls*	3 and 10		

*With elastic bands

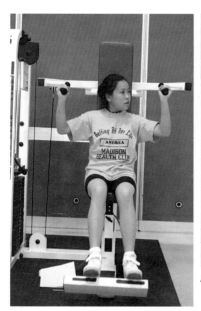

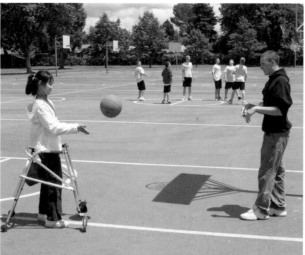

A good activity plan includes a variety of different activities.

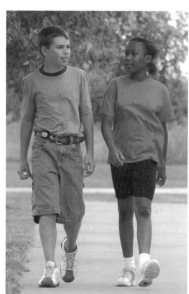

Biomechanical Principles: Integration

Efficient performance in physical activities is often complicated and requires you to apply several biomechanical principles at the same time.

In the previous chapters you learned about eight different biomechanical principles. You learned how to apply these principles to help you perform more efficiently and effectively in sports and physical activities of all kinds. **Integration** means combining several different things into one whole thing. Integrating several biomechanical principles means applying several of them at the same time to make one whole movement more efficient and effective.

Playing a sport requires several different types of movements. Different principles are used in performing each of these movements. For example, in playing a sport such as basketball, you need offensive skills such as shooting, dribbling, catching, and passing. You must apply the principles of biomechanics relating to energy and force, levers, and friction in order to have a good performance. When playing defense, you must have stability and range of motion, and you must know how to use friction. Each skill requires that you integrate several principles to have a good performance.

Applying the Principle

Think about the biomechanical principles that you have studied: energy, force, and movement; levers; friction; stability and balance; velocity, acceleration, and deceleration; range of motion; resistance; and efficiency. Now, consider how you integrate the principles in different activities.

For example, to stop a penalty kick, a soccer goalie must stand in a balanced position but be ready to move with great force very quickly. She often jumps or dives into the air while judging the flight path of the ball, and she reaches with several levers to block the shot. Her ability to jump sideways depends on friction between her shoes and the ground and the relationship of her base to her center of gravity when she pushes off.

Consider a swimmer as another example. He must have plenty of energy and muscular endurance. He uses the levers of his arms and legs to push against the water. A large range of motion in his shoulders helps create the most effective arm stroke. He moves in ways that create as little resistance as possible because resistance slows his body down.

Describe how the following activities require the integration of several principles:

► Tennis
► Golf
► Baseball
► Walking

Principles in Practice

When performing physical activities of all kinds, you must integrate several principles to prepare for good performance. Identify two skills used in an activity that you enjoy. For example, if you enjoy playing soccer, you might choose running and kicking. Then determine how you can perform one of these two skills more effectively by applying the principles that you have learned. Practice the skill using the new information.

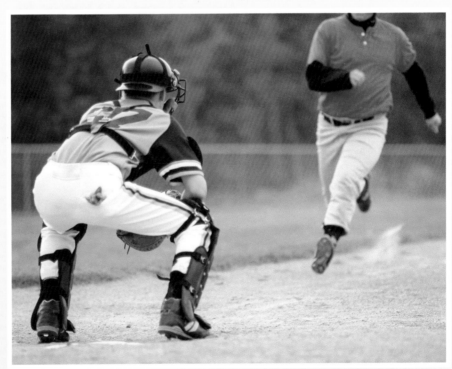

Baseball players need stability, use body levers, apply force, and use other principles to perform well.

© Photodisc

Click Student Info ► Topic 9.6

During the first four weeks of the summer, Keisha performed her plan. She kept an activity log that included making check marks for each activity that she performed each day. Keisha missed a few of her activity sessions on a few days, but she was able to make up for the misses by doing the activities on other days. At the end of four weeks, Keisha had met her short-term activity goals because she had regularly performed her activity plan. Putting your plan in writing helps you stick with it.

Keisha was encouraged by her success and decided to use the same short-term goals and follow the same activity plan for another four weeks. Because she had been active for a while, Keisha decided to add long-term fitness goals to her plan (see table 9.7). She set the long-term fitness goals of reaching the healthy fitness zone for each of the Fitnessgram tests by the end of the summer.

Keisha met her activity goals again for the second four weeks of the summer. She then did a follow-up assessment using Fitnessgram. She improved her fitness and met her long-term goal of reaching the healthy fitness zone for all of the Fitnessgram self-assessments.

You can follow the same steps that Keisha followed. You can

1. do a fitness summary,
2. do a physical activity summary,
3. set SMART goals,
4. write a physical activity plan,
5. keep an activity log to determine whether you met your short-term goals, and
6. after meeting several short-term goals, assess your long-term goals.

Your teacher will provide you with the worksheets necessary to follow these six steps. You'll get a chance to try some of the activities in your plan in class. But if you're going to be as successful as Keisha was, it will be important for you to be active outside of class as well. Your support team can help you to develop and carry out your plan.

Table 9.7

Keisha's Long-Term Fitness Goals

Type of fitness	Long-term fitness goals
Cardiovascular fitness	Maintain current fitness in the healthy fitness zone.*
Flexibility	Improve sit-and-reach score to reach the healthy fitness zone.*
Muscle fitness	Improve curl-up and push-up scores to reach the healthy fitness zone.*
Body composition	Maintain body fatness and BMI in the healthy fitness zone.*

*Keisha added these long-term goals after the first four weeks of working on her short-term activity goals. To meet her long-term goals, she kept the same activity goals as listed in table 9.5.

Lesson Review

▶ What are some steps that you can follow in setting SMART goals?

▶ What is the difference between a short-term goal and a long-term goal?

▶ Describe the steps you take in developing a personal activity plan.

▶ How is integration important to performance in physical activity?

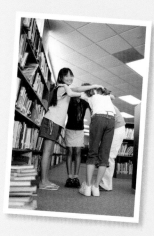

9 Chapter Review

Number your paper from 1 to 5. Read each question. After the number for the question, write a word or a phrase that best answers the question. The page number where you can find the answer is listed after the question.

1. What is the name of the report that gives the results of all fitness tests a person has performed? (page 105)
2. What is the name of the report that gives the results of all physical activities a person performs each week? (page 106)
3. What kind of goal can be accomplished in a few days or weeks? (page 110)
4. What five-letter word can help you remember the factors that make up good goals? (page 111)
5. What word means combining different biomechanical principles to make performance more efficient? (page 113)

Number your paper from 6 to 10. Next to each number, write the letter of the best answer.

6. flexibility activities   a. teens who get no regular activity
7. long term   b. goals that take months to accomplish
8. 12 percent   c. level 3 of the Physical Activity Pyramid
9. Keisha   d. teen who built an activity plan
10. lifestyle activities   e. level 1 of the Physical Activity Pyramid

Number your paper from 11 to 15. Follow the directions to answer each question or statement.

11. What is a fitness summary, and what information should it include?
12. What is a physical activity summary, and what information should it include?
13. Give examples of guidelines that can help you become fit and active.
14. Explain how each letter in SMART can help you set goals for activity.
15. What is integration, and how is it important to using biomechanical principles in activity?

Ask the Authors

Why do some kids who don't do a lot of exercise score better on fitness tests than other kids who exercise a lot?

Get the answer and ask your own questions at the *Fitness for Life: Middle School* Web site.

Click Student Info ▶ Topic 9.7

Unit Review on the Web

You can find unit III review materials on the *Fitness for Life: Middle School* Web site.

Click Student Info ▶ Topic 9.8

glossary

The terms in this glossary have many different meanings depending on the circumstances in which they're used. In this glossary the terms are defined so that they're appropriate for use in middle school physical education classes in a variety of physical activities.

A

acceleration—An increase in the speed (velocity) of a movement.

active aerobics—Continuous, vigorous activities that get the heart beating fast enough to build cardiovascular fitness; for example, jogging, aerobic dance.

active recreation—Recreational activities that are vigorous enough to increase the heart rate enough to build cardiovascular fitness.

active sports—Sports that are vigorous enough to increase the heart rate enough to build cardiovascular fitness.

aerobic—"With oxygen"; activity is aerobic when the body can supply enough oxygen to keep going for long periods of time.

agility—The ability to change body positions quickly and keep the body under control when moving.

anaerobic—"Without oxygen"; in this book it refers to activities for which the body can't supply enough oxygen to keep going for long periods of time (for example, sprinting).

B

balance—The ability to keep the body in a steady position while standing or moving.

ballistic stretching—Exercises that cause muscles and tendons to get longer than normal; caused by movements such as bouncing or bobbing.

basal metabolism—A term used to describe the amount of energy the body expends when in an inactive or basic (basal) state.

body composition—The combination of all of the tissues that make up the body such as bones, muscles, organs, and body fat.

body fatness—The percentage of total body weight that is composed of fat.

body image—A person's feelings about his or her body; a good body image requires positive feelings about one's body, including feelings about the way one looks.

body mass index (BMI)—A formula that determines a healthy body weight based on height.

C

calipers—An instrument used to measure thickness; skinfold calipers measure the thickness of fat folds beneath the skin.

calories—A unit of measure for energy; in this book it refers to the energy contained in foods. For example, a soft drink with sugar typically contains 150 calories.

carbohydrates—Substances in food that provide energy; sugars and starches.

cardiovascular fitness—The ability of the heart, lungs, blood vessels, and blood to work efficiently and to supply the body with oxygen.

CDC—The abbreviation for the Centers for Disease Control and Prevention, a government agency dedicated to promoting good health among United States citizens.

center of gravity—The center of your body weight.

cool-down—Exercise designed to help you recover after physical activity; includes cardiovascular activity followed by stretching exercises.

coordination—The ability of body parts to work together when you perform an activity.

cramp—An involuntary contraction of a muscle that can be painful.

D

deceleration—A reduction in velocity or speed.

discretionary foods—A term used in MyPyramid for foods that do not fit in any single category such as fruits, vegetables, meats, and milk products; refers to foods such as ketchup, mustard, and sauces used with other foods.

E

eating disorder—A dangerous (and potentially life-threatening) condition associated with eating too little and often exercising too much.

efficiency—the ability to perform with little wasted energy or wasted time.

energy—Available power; in this book it refers to the power available to cause the body's muscles to contract.

energy balance—Taking in the same number of calories (energy intake) as you expend (energy expenditure).

energy expenditure—The calories that the body expends in performing its normal functions and physical activities.

energy intake—The calories one consumes from food.

essential fat—The minimum percentage of body fat that is necessary to have good health.

exercise—Activity designed to build one or more of the health-related parts of physical fitness.

F

fats—Oily substances in food from animal and plant sources that provide energy and that are necessary for other bodily functions.

feedback—Information from an instructor or another source that helps one change a performance or a skill.

first-class levers—A type of lever in which the fulcrum (or pivot point) is between the resistance (or weight) and the effort (or force), such as a seesaw or the foot when walking.

Fitnessgram—A national fitness test that includes tests for all parts of health-related fitness.

fitness summary—A chart or table that describes (summarizes) a person's fitness for every part of health-related fitness; useful as a basis for setting personal goals and in creating a physical activity plan.

FITT—A collection of letters (acronym) used to describe the formula for building fitness: F for frequency, I for intensity, T for time, and T for type.

flexibility—The ability to move all body parts and joints freely.

flexibility exercises—A type of physical activity designed to build flexibility by stretching the muscles (and tendons) longer than normal.

flexion—A movement that reduces the angle of a joint; for example, when you flex the elbow, the angle of the lower arm and the upper arm gets smaller.

force—In this book force refers to a cause of body movement resulting from the contraction of the muscles.

friction—Resistance to motion caused by one surface rubbing against another.

G

games—Activities that have simple rules and often a winner or loser, but that may or may not require the use of the large muscles. Capture the flag is an active game; computer games are inactive games.

gravity—The force that causes objects to fall toward earth.

H

health-related fitness—One of two general categories of physical fitness (the other is skill-related physical fitness). The five parts of health-related fitness (body composition, cardiovascular fitness, flexibility, muscular endurance, and strength) are associated with good health.

healthy fitness zone—The amount of fitness a person needs to be healthy.

hypermobility—Too much range of motion in a joint; also called joint laxity.

I

integration—Putting several parts together to make a whole; in this book it refers to using several biomechanical principles together to produce efficient and effective movement.

isometric exercises—A type of physical activity (exercise) in which the body parts don't move, such as pushing the arms together in front of the body so that the force produced in each arm is equal.

isotonic exercise—A type of physical activity (exercise) in which the body parts move, such as push-ups and resistance exercises with weights or machines.

J

joint—The place in the body where two or more bones are connected, such as the elbow.

L

lever—A bar or stiff, straight object (simple machine) used to lift weight, produce force, or create speed.

lifestyle physical activities—Physical activities that are moderate in intensity and are used in normal daily activity.

lifetime activities—Physical activities, including sports, that can be done throughout life; examples include golf, tennis, jogging, and resistance training.

lifetime sports—A sport such as golf or tennis that can be played by people of all ages.

ligaments—Body tissues that connect bones to bones.

long-term goals—Objectives that can require many weeks or months to achieve.

M

mental practice—Rehearsing a skill in one's mind (imagining a performance) in an attempt to improve a skill or performance.

minerals—Substances in food that come from plants or animal sources; examples include calcium, salt, and potassium.

moderate activities—Physical activities that are equal in intensity to brisk walking. When done with enough frequency and intensity and for a long enough time, moderate activity has many health benefits.

motor skills—Another name for skills; in this book, it refers to the use of the nerves and muscles together.

motor units—Groups of nerves and muscle cells that work together to produce movement and allow people to perform skills.

muscle(s)—Body tissue that lengthens and shortens to cause movement of the bones that results in body movement; tissue that contracts without movement to support the body and hold objects.

muscle fitness—A type of health-related fitness; includes strength and muscular endurance.

muscle fitness exercises—A type of physical activity that is designed to build strength, muscular endurance, or both; examples include calisthenics, push-ups, and weight-lifting.

muscular endurance—The ability to use muscles for a long period of time without getting tired.

MyPyramid—A diagram prepared by the United States Department of Agriculture to help people understand the many nutrients necessary in a healthy diet.

N

NASPE—An abbreviation for the National Association for Sport and Physical Education.

nutrients—The things we eat (foods) and the substances included in food; examples include carbohydrates, proteins, fats, vitamins, minerals, and water.

O

osteoporosis—A condition that occurs when the bones lose strength and become weak and brittle.

overweight—Having more body weight than is desirable for good health.

P

PACER—Initials used for the Fitnessgram test of cardiovascular fitness; the letters stand for progressive aerobic cardiovascular endurance run.

paralysis by analysis—A condition that can harm skill performance, occurring when you get so much information about your performance that you can't use it all.

participation sports—Sports that require a person to be active (participation) as opposed to being a watcher (spectator).

PCPFS—An abbreviation for the President's Council on Physical Fitness and Sports; a U.S. government agency dedicated to promoting fitness and physical activity.

pedometer—A small computer worn on the belt that counts the steps taken in physical activity.

performance skills—Skills performed in a variety of settings such as sports and work.

physical activity—Movement that uses the large muscles of the body, including sports, lifestyle activities, active aerobics and recreation, dance, and fitness exercises.

physical activity summary—A chart or table that describes (summarizes) a person's current level of activity in all of the types of activity described in the Physical Activity Pyramid; useful as a basis for setting personal goals and creating a physical activity plan.

physical fitness—The ability of the body systems to work together efficiently.

physical recreation—Activities done during free time that use the large muscles of the body, such as playing tag, fishing, or hiking.

PNF (proprioceptive neuromuscular facilitation)—A type of static stretch that requires the muscle to be contracted immediately before it is stretched.

power—The ability to combine strength with speed while moving.

practice—Repeating an action over and over to improve skill.

principle of overload—A rule that states that one must do more physical activity than normal to build fitness; for example, doing muscle exercise to build muscle fitness.

principle of progression—A rule that states that overload must be gradual to be the most beneficial.

progressive resistance exercise (PRE)—Exercise that gradually overloads the muscles of the body to produce fitness.

protein—Substance in food that provides energy and is necessary for building body tissues; sources include meats, beans, nuts, and milk products.

R

range of motion—The amount of movement in a joint.

reaction time—The ability to move quickly once a signal to start moving is received.

recreation—Activities done during free time; they may be relatively active or inactive.

rep—A short term for repetition (see *repetition*).

repetition—Each instance that a person performs (repeats) an exercise.

resistance—Opposition to a force or a movement.

resting heart rate—The number of times the heart beats per minute during rest; to determine this number, take your heart rate when you first get up in the morning.

routine—Performing movements in the same way time after time; a technique used to enhance skill performance.

S

second-class levers—A type of lever in which the weight (or resistance) is between the fulcrum (or pivot point) and the effort (or force), such as a wheelbarrow.

sedentary—A term used to describe a person who does no regular physical activity.

self-esteem—A person's feelings about himself or herself; good self-esteem requires positive feelings about oneself.

set—Groups of repetitions of an exercise; for example, performing 10 repetitions followed by a rest is one set.

short-term goals—Objectives that can be achieved in a few days or up to several weeks.

skill—The capacity to perform a specific task that involves the use of the muscles and nerves together with the brain.

skill-related fitness—One of two general categories of physical fitness (the other is health-related physical fitness); the six parts of skill-related fitness (agility, balance, coordination, power, speed, and reaction time) are associated with the ability to learn skills and perform well in certain activities and jobs.

SMART goals—A collection of letters (acronym) that describes the qualities of good goals: S is for specific, M is for measurable, A is for attainable, R is for reasonable, and T is for timely.

specificity—A rule or principle that states that you must overload the specific system of the body that you want to improve; for example, doing curl-ups will improve your abdominal muscles but not your cardiovascular system.

spectator sports—Sports such as football that people watch rather than perform regularly.

speed—The ability to get from one place to another in the shortest possible time.

sports—Physical activities that have rules and winners and losers and that involve competition; for example, football and tennis.

sport skills—The ability to perform specific tasks required to play sports, such as kicking, throwing, and catching.

stability—The ability to maintain balance.

static stretching—Exercises that cause muscles and tendons to get longer than normal; these stretches require the person to hold the muscle in the lengthened position for a period of time.

strain—An injury to a muscle; a tear in muscle tissue.

strategy—A comprehensive plan to do one's best in a game or sport; a strategy often involves combining several tactics, such as using a zone defense.

strength—The ability of muscles to lift a heavy weight or exert a lot of force.

supplements—Defined by the Food and Drug Administration as a product taken by mouth that contains a "dietary ingredient" intended to supplement the diet.

T

tactics—Decisions to use one's skills to best advantage in a game or sport; for example, moving quickly to an open spot to receive a pass.

target zone—A phrase used to describe the intensity of an activity that is necessary to promote a benefit such as fitness improvement. Each type of activity from the Physical Activity Pyramid has its own target zone.

tendons—Body tissues that connect muscles to bones.

third-class levers—A type of lever in which the effort (or force applied) is between the weight (or resistance) and the fulcrum (or pivot point), such as the arm throwing a ball or the leg kicking a ball.

V

velocity—The speed of a movement.

vigorous activities—Physical activities that are intense enough to cause the heart to beat faster than normal and that build cardiovascular fitness.

vitamins—Substances contained in food that are necessary for normal growth and development as well as good health; examples include vitamins A, B, C, D, and E. Vitamins can be obtained in pills or capsules as well as in food.

W

warm-up—Exercise designed to get you ready for physical activity; includes cardiovascular activity followed by stretching exercises.

muscle fitness
  benefits of 85-86, 85*f*, 90
  defined 79
  exercises for 79-80, 81*t*, 82
  factors affecting 88
  Physical Activity Pyramid and 4
  ratings for 86-87, 88*t*
  supplements and 84
muscle groups 90, 90*f*
muscular endurance 9, 79
MyPyramid 99-100, 99*f*

N

NASCAR auto racing 19
National Association for Sport and Physical
    Activity (NASPE) 28
negative comments 43
Newton's laws of motion 11
noncompetitive activities 68
nutrients 99
nutrition 99-100, 99*f*

O

osteoporosis 85
outdoor recreation activities 55, 55*t*
overfat, defined 94
overload, principle of 79
overweight, health risks of 94

P

PACER test 47, 50, 50*t*
paralysis by analysis 24
PAR-Q questionnaire 30
participation sports 53
partner-assisted stretch 67*f*
PCPFS (President's Council on Physical Fitness
    and Sports) 29
pedometer 29
peer pressure 97
performance, comparisons of 42
performance skills 16
personal information, confidentiality of 43,
    95
personal strengths 42
persons with disabilities 55

physical activity
  benefits of 6
  defined 3
  energy balance and 99-100, 102
  safety during 30, 47, 80
  types of 3-4
  warming up and cooling down for 6, 6*f*, 30
physical activity needs 105-109, 110, 111*t*
physical activity plan 108, 111, 112*t*, 114
Physical Activity Pyramid 3, 4*f*, 5*f*, 29
physical activity summary 106-107, 106*t*
physical fitness. *See also* cardiovascular fitness;
    muscle fitness; skill-related fitness
  assessment of 10, 12. *See also* Fitnessgram
  components of 9-10
  defined 9
  health-related 9, 9*f*
  heredity and 12
  lifestyle physical activities and 35
physical recreation. *See* active recreation
PNF (proprioceptive neuromuscular facilita-
    tion) 66
positive thinking 42
posture
  flexibility and 71, 71*f*
  muscle fitness and 85, 85*f*
power 17*t*
practice 16, 20, 20*f*, 24, 24*f*
PRE (progressive resistance exercise) 79-80
President's Council on Physical Fitness and
    Sports (PCPFS) 29
principle of overload 79
principle of progression 80
privacy of personal information 43, 95
progression, principle of 80
Progressive Aerobic Cardiovascular Endurance
    Run (PACER) 47, 50, 50*t*
progressive resistance exercise (PRE) 79-80
proprioceptive neuromuscular facilitation
    (PNF) 66
protective gear 30
proteins, dietary 100
pulse 40*f*
push-up test 86

R

range of motion 65, 73-74
reaction time 17*t*